Marissa Henley has written us who have friends struggl ... the first place I'll go as I seek to care for people with not only cancer, but any serious illness. Marissa's practical helps are worth the price of the book.

— **Dave Furman**, senior pastor, Redeemer Church of Dubai; author, *Being There: How to Love Those Who Are Hurting* and *Kiss the Wave: Embracing God in Your Trials*

This immanently practical book gives gospel-infused advice from a fellow pilgrim who has been shepherded through the valley of the shadow of death. Marissa calls the body of Christ to engage head, heart, and hands for the purpose of coming alongside those who are suffering.

— **Karen Hodge**, PCA women's ministry coordinator

Marissa reminds us that the One who created us has not abandoned our friend—or us. Our friend's cancer diagnosis provides an opportunity for us to gently move toward them, share the love of Christ by being his hands and feet, and enter into their suffering in the same way Jesus entered into ours. It is a journey worth taking, and this book is an excellent travel guide.

— **Brian Holt**, president and CEO, Hope Cancer Resources

When you walk beside someone with the life-changing diagnosis of cancer, knowing what to do and say is so difficult. As a professional counselor, I am excited for people in that position to have the honest perspective that Marissa brings to these difficult circumstances. And on a personal note, as someone who has lost three family members to cancer over the past three years, I wish I'd had this book to share with our community.

— **Michelle Nietert**, clinical director, Community Counseling Associates; Counselor Thoughts podcaster; speaker; author

Anyone who's been touched by cancer, to any degree, will be helped and comforted by this beautiful book. Marissa addresses a difficult, life-changing battle with eloquence, truth, and intense practicality, inviting us into her cancer story and to the God who is her hope. I see Jesus in Marissa as she proclaims him through her sufferings, and I pray he will equip many readers through her wise counsel in these pages.

—**Kristen Wetherell**, coauthor, *Hope When It Hurts: Biblical Reflections to Help You Grasp God's Purpose in Your Suffering*

LOVING
YOUR
FRIEND
THROUGH
CANCER

LOVING YOUR FRIEND THROUGH CANCER

Moving beyond "I'm Sorry"
to Meaningful Support

MARISSA HENLEY

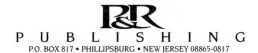

P&R PUBLISHING
P.O. BOX 817 • PHILLIPSBURG • NEW JERSEY 08865-0817

Printed in the United States of America

Library of Congress Cataloging-in-Publication Data

Names: Henley, Marissa, author.
Title: Loving your friend through cancer : moving beyond I'm sorry to meaningful support / Marissa Henley.
Description: Phillipsburg : P&R Publishing, 2018. | Includes bibliographical references and index.
Identifiers: LCCN 2018002006| ISBN 9781629953540 (pbk.) | ISBN 9781629953557 (epub) | ISBN 9781629953564 (mobi)
Subjects: LCSH: Cancer--Religious aspects--Christianity. | Cancer--Patients--Religious life. | Friendship--Religious aspects--Christianity. | Caring--Religious aspects--Christianity.
Classification: LCC BV4910.33 .H46 2018 | DDC 248.8/6196994--dc23
LC record available at https://lccn.loc.gov/2018002006

To my friends,

who battled cancer with me,
walk through survivorship with me,
and teach me by example how to love others with cancer.

The evil that hurts us now will be the
eventual servant of our joy and glory eternally.
—Tim Keller, in Be Still, My Soul

Contents

Contents

Resources

Preface

The phone rings, and your heart stops. You look down at the screen and see the name of your dear friend who has been waiting for biopsy results. As your shaking fingers fumble to answer the call, your heart cries out a silent prayer.

You immediately hear the shock and sadness in her voice. You know even before she utters the words. "It's cancer."

On a Monday afternoon in October 2010, my friends and family received this phone call from me. I was an energetic mom of three young children and never imagined that by Thanksgiving I would be incapable of caring for my family. As I battled cancer for the next nine months, my friends shouldered the responsibility of all that I was suddenly powerless to do. They cared for my home and my family, and they ministered to my heart and soul. In fact, they should be the ones writing this book. They are the true experts. But I think they may still be playing catch-up from the time they spent running my life back then, so they left the book-writing up to me.

As a cancer survivor, I hear this question often: "A friend of mine was just diagnosed with cancer. How can I help? How do I support her? I'm so afraid I'll do or say the wrong thing!" Since you're reading this, you're probably asking these same questions. I wish we could sit down over a cup of coffee and talk face-to-face. I'd ask you about your friend. I'd ask you about her family, her treatment, and her unique challenges.

We would sip our lattes and you'd tell me how heartbroken you are for her. My eyes would fill with tears, because I've been there—as the one with cancer, but also as the friend wondering how to help.

These pages contain the conversation I wish we could have about your friend—what she's experiencing and how you can support her. I'm eager to introduce you to several of my cancer-surviving friends and to share the stories of how their friends supported them through their illness and survivorship. I hope their stories will expand on my own to give you a richer understanding of the experience of cancer.

In addition to the practical information you'll find in each chapter, I've included resources at the back of the book that explore the biblical foundations of suffering and community. Our beliefs drive our behavior, even as we care for those with cancer. We are the body of Christ, and caring for the sick is a responsibility we should approach with thoughtfulness and intentionality. As we live in community and love those with cancer, even the support that we provide is done in community with others. You are not alone in this tough assignment of supporting your friend through cancer. I'm grateful to be on your team!

If you're looking for the short version, I'd tell you to be there for your friend for the long haul, ask questions instead of making assumptions, listen to her, and love her well. But if you want to dig deeper, keep reading. As you read the stories and suggestions, please remember that every person is different, every family is different, and every cancer is different. My hope for the guidance and examples I share within these pages is that they will help you develop your own plan to care for your friend. (You'll find questions at the end of each chapter to help you apply what you're learning to your friend's unique situation.) Together, we will equip you to be a better friend.

We will broaden your perspective on life-threatening illnesses. And we will prepare your heart to respond with love to your friend's suffering.

Your friend's situation is unique, so remember to approach her as a unique person. If she's fiercely independent and stubborn, make gentle offers of assistance and be patient. If relationships energize her, arrange a lunch out with friends to lift her spirits. If she cherishes order and organization, perhaps you can love her best by cleaning and organizing her pantry or kids' closets. Consider honestly the closeness of your friendship with her, and be careful not to force a level of intimacy with your offers of help that might make her uncomfortable. (Chapter 2 provides guidelines for this.)

My purpose in this book is not to convince you to take the burden off your friend's back and place it on your own. You will not be able to meet all her needs. You are just one link in the chain of support that God is assembling around her. Please avoid the temptation to view this book as a to-do list. Although I hope it will give ideas that you can use and share with others, you cannot do everything mentioned in this book. If you begin to feel overwhelmed, turn to chapter 3 and read more about how you won't be doing everything for your friend. Take the suggestions in this book and add your own prayers for wisdom and your unique knowledge of your friend, and you will be ready to walk compassionately beside your friend through her illness.

Acknowledgments

Writing a book is not an individual sport. You would not be holding this book in your hands if it weren't for my team of family, friends, cheerleaders, interviewees, and professionals. So, before we go any further, I'd like to thank them for getting us to this point.

Thank you to Amanda Martin and Kristi James at P&R Publishing for your editorial expertise and encouragement. I appreciate your patience with me as a first-time author with lots of questions. Thank you to Ann Kroeker for your invaluable coaching during the writing process. I wouldn't have wanted to tackle this project without your wisdom and gentle prodding toward the finish line. Thank you to my pastor, Hunter Bailey, for your insights on a biblical view of suffering. And thank you to Callie Granderson for taking an author photograph that makes me smile.

To the fighters, survivors, and caregivers who shared their cancer experiences with me, some of whom are mentioned by name in these pages and others of whom contributed to the principles and suggestions I give: Crystal, Bev, Samantha, Becky, Lisa, Debbie, Liz, Jamie, Kristi, Marilyn, Anna, Alexis, Ashley, Courtney, Jess, Pam, Aimee, John, Sara, Mary, Billy, Ed, Marni, Lesley, Karen, Lisa, and Janet. Thank you for trusting me with your stories. I hope I have stewarded them well.

To Amanda, Ashley, Courtney, Erin, Jenny, Jessica, Lynette,

Mandy, Maria, Marilyn, Susan, my Voxer friends, my parents, and many other friends and family members who cheered me on and asked repeatedly, "How's the book?": your prayers and encouragement are worth more than gold.

To my kids: Thank you for sharing me with this project and for having total confidence in my efforts. I pray that someday you use the gifts God's given you for his glory and for the good of his kingdom.

To my husband, Noel, who endured sub-par dinners, unfolded laundry, and an extremely distracted wife for months while I wrote this manuscript: You never doubted whether or not this was a good idea, even when I did. Thank you for being my most amazing supporter.

To my friends and family who walked with me through cancer and the years following: You know who you are, and you know how much I love you. You built a beautiful house of selfless compassion in my life with Christ as the foundation. In this book, I have simply cut a window in the wall to let others look in and see what you've done. By blessing me, you are now blessing others. It's an honor to be your friend.

To God alone be the glory.

Introduction

I'm so sorry you picked up this book. Can we start there? Let's begin by acknowledging the reason you're reading this. Your loved one has cancer, or you have cancer—or you fear you've made friendship mistakes in the past and you want to be prepared next time, because you know cancer won't stay away from your circle of friends for long. I desperately wish no one ever needed to read this book—I *hate* cancer. But until we cure cancer or Jesus returns, we need to struggle through this together. We need information, ideas, prayer, strength, and free-flowing forgiveness as we seek to support our friends with cancer.

I wish I could go back and talk to my 2010 self. I would sit down across from a frightened, bald young mom as the chemo dripped into her veins. I'd show her pictures from 2017, when she has hair past her shoulders and kids who are old enough to remember the memories she's making with them. I'd tell her that she will be raising a teenager, enjoying her forties, and writing a book. She would never believe me. She'd laugh in disbelief to hear that she will parasail for her fortieth birthday, watch her son star in the school musical, and even cave when her kids beg for a puppy. If I told her all that, she would never believe me. In that moment, she was just hanging on from day to day. I wish she could know what was yet to come.

As much as I'd love to visit my 2010 self, I'd like even more to visit my 2009 self. She stands by the kitchen sink with her face in her hands, absorbing the news of her sister-in-law's breast cancer diagnosis. As two preschool-age boys run around her and the newborn wakes from a nap, she wonders how she can possibly help. How can she serve? What should she say? What should she not say? She has no clue.

My 2009 self got some of it right. She organized meals. She took care of her two-year-old niece on Fridays to give other family members a reprieve. She checked on her sister-in-law regularly and tried to offer words of comfort.

My 2009 self also got a lot of it wrong. I would love to go back and tell 2009 Marissa to shut her mouth and listen more. I'd tell her to stop using Bible verses to dismiss her sister-in-law's pain. To stop trying to talk her out of being scared. And to *please* stop comparing chemo-related nausea and fatigue to that which she experienced during her recent, healthy pregnancy.

One problem that 2009 Marissa faced was that she didn't understand what her sister-in-law was experiencing. I'd like to think that if my sister-in-law had been diagnosed in 2011, after I had gained firsthand knowledge of what cancer feels like, my support would have shown more compassion and creativity, as well as offering practical and emotional solutions, because it would have flowed from a better understanding of what truly helps.

Even today I make missteps. Words sometimes pop out of my mouth without enough forethought, and I wish I could take them back. And everyone is different—words and actions that helped and supported me might not be what another person truly wants or needs. But it is definitely easier to know how to love and support someone going through cancer when you've walked that road yourself. I have. And I'm here to share with you my best ideas and solutions.

If you are a friend seeking to love someone with cancer,

I hope this book will be a great substitute for firsthand experience. I want to pull back the curtain and show you what it feels like to have cancer and what your friend needs. I was a young mom when I had cancer, but you'll find information in this book that is relevant to all ages and stages. If you're a survivor who wants to learn more, I'm ready with stories from several cancer-fighters and caregivers that will give you fresh ideas. If you're a cancer-fighter or caregiver who needs to make sense of what you're feeling and experiencing, I wrote this book for you, too. Whatever your reason for picking up this book, I pray that it ministers to you and encourages you.

Cancer is a painful topic, and I've taken care to write with sensitivity. Unfortunately, addressing this subject adequately requires touching on subjects relating to medical procedures, hospitalization, illness, end-of-life care, and even death. Some of these topics may be particularly difficult for you to read about. I wish it didn't have to be that way. Before one copy of this book was printed, I prayed Romans 15:13 for you: "May the God of hope fill you with all joy and peace in believing, so that by the power of the Holy Spirit you may abound in hope." As we push through these hard topics together, I'm in this with you. And, more importantly, the power of the Holy Spirit will fill you with joy and hope. He will hold us fast as we enter the storm of suffering.

When Cancer
Strikes a Friendship

Facing Your New Assignment

The Phone Call

When I describe my cancer experience, October 25, 2010, is the day I share in the most detail—because those are the details I will never forget. I had just finished giving instructions to a babysitter before leaving for a parent-teacher conference at my first-grader's school. My phone rang, and I saw that it was the radiologist who had biopsied the lump in my breast a few days earlier.

I hurried to my bedroom to answer the call. As I stood by my bed, I heard the doctor say, "I'm sorry, Marissa; this is a tumor." He explained that it wasn't breast cancer but rather cancer in the lining of the blood vessels—a rare and aggressive cancer called angiosarcoma. I sat on the edge of the bed and searched in my nightstand for a paper and pen. I'd never heard this strange word before and needed him to spell it. As he explained more, I rushed to the computer and typed it into Google. But my mind was too shocked to read anything on the screen. Concerned by my silence, the doctor asked if I was okay. I said, "I'm not sure if you're telling me I have one year, or five years, or what." His reply was not reassuring: "We just don't know yet."

It was the day before my thirty-fourth birthday. My boys were ages six and four, and my baby girl was not yet eighteen months old. And, when I ended the call with the doctor and turned my attention to the computer screen, I read that only 30 percent of those diagnosed with this disease live for five years. I slammed my laptop shut. The first of many tears began falling as I begged the Lord to let me walk my baby into first grade. It was my earnest prayer for months and then years, and still is today: "Lord, please let me live to see my babies grow up. Please, Lord. Please."

In my shock and grief, the Lord poured out comfort and peace through his Word and through the prayers and encouragement of others. Two weeks after my diagnosis, I wrote about that difficult day in my online CaringBridge journal:

> That afternoon is kind of a blur. I remember during one of the early phone calls, I was starting to lose it and just started repeating out loud, 'God is good. God is good. God is good.' All I could do in those first terrible moments was to cling to what I knew to be true about God. I knew that everything I had known to be true about His character, His power, His love for me and His faithfulness were still just as true as it had been hours before. I knew from what we had been studying in Isaiah that God had given me this assignment for His glory and for my good. Because I belong to God in Christ, nothing can separate me from His love.

Due to the rare and aggressive nature of the cancer, I received treatment at MD Anderson Cancer Center in Houston, Texas, six hundred miles from my hometown. The first step in my nine-month treatment plan was high doses of chemotherapy. Every three weeks, I received four straight days of chemo, including a pump that I wore around the clock. The first two rounds took place in my hometown. After those initial rounds, a CT scan showed significant shrinking of the tumor. This was great news for my long-term prognosis. If chemo shrank the tumor, then we could hope it was destroying lingering cancer cells that could metastasize in the future.

But then we learned that I needed to enroll in a clinical trial to receive the rest of the chemo, and I started spending two out of every three weeks in Houston. At that time, I wasn't sure I would live long enough for my daughter to remember me. I didn't want to spend any of the time I had left in a Houston hospital room. But I didn't have a choice. I spent nine weeks away from my family and missed New Year's, Valentine's Day, and all three of my kids' birthdays. The logistical challenges were daunting. And yet the Lord provided for every need, and my friends pitched in both in Houston and at home to care for us. (You'll read all about their kindness and support in the following chapters—I can't wait to tell you more!)

When I was home, I was usually weak and sick, requiring several blood transfusions and dealing with complications from having low red blood cells, white blood cells, and platelets. I needed countless injections, blood draws, and medications. I visited some sort of health care facility almost every day, with no hair, no eyebrows, no eyelashes, and a central line coming out of my chest.

After seven rounds of chemo, the tumor had shrunk to almost nothing, and my body couldn't take any more of the harsh drugs. The next step was radiation: five days a week for five weeks, in Houston. I hated spending more time away from home, but I felt much better physically. We brought the kids to Houston for two weeks and explored the city together. It was almost like a family vacation, except for the time each day when I lay inside a machine and had a high-energy beam of radiation shot at my life-threatening tumor.

Following radiation, I returned home for several weeks. My hometown doctors struggled to get my platelets, which were still devastated from chemo, high enough for me to have surgery. In July 2011, I returned to Houston for a mastectomy. The Lord used the skilled hands of my surgeon to remove the last traces of cancer from my body with widely clear margins.

And then, ten months after that phone call, I heard a cancer survivor's four favorite words: "No evidence of disease." By God's grace, I remain cancer-free today.

My Friends Carried My Load

My friends began caring for me within hours of my diagnosis. One friend folded laundry in my bedroom while I made endless phone calls, and another friend silently cooked spaghetti in my kitchen. We were all in shock.

In the days that followed, I kept apologizing to my friends. I knew they were distraught and their lives would be challenging in the coming months. The year before, I had walked the road of cancer with my sister-in-law, and I knew the sacrifices that would be required of my friends. Finally, one of my best friends sat me down and said, "Marissa, you keep telling us this is an assignment for you from the Lord. Well, he didn't give this assignment only to you. He gave us this assignment, too. We are ready. We are in this with you. So stop apologizing to us."

Over the next several months, my friends sacrificed and suffered with me. Sometimes one of them refers to that time as "when we had cancer," and then tries to correct herself by saying, "I mean, when you had cancer." And every time, I tell her, "No, we had cancer together."

God repeatedly showed us he was going to meet each and every one of our needs, just as he had promised. He placed us in a caring community in the town where my husband and I were born and raised. He surrounded us with a wide circle of loving friends through our church family, our neighbors, my husband's colleagues, our parents' churches, and a small Christian school that acted like another church family. He used an army of friends, family, acquaintances, and even strangers to provide tangible, emotional, and spiritual support as we battled for my health and for my life. Every time our challenges seemed insurmountable, the Lord revealed the next step in his plan to provide for us.

None of my friends could meet all my needs, but they each did what they could. They brought meals to our family three nights a week for eight months. They drove my kids to school, preschool, piano lessons, and play dates. They traveled to Houston to care for me during chemo. They put my name on prayer lists all over the country. They sent texts, emails, and cards to remind me I was loved. They listened compassionately as I struggled with grief, anger, fear, and stress. God wove my friends' threads of support into a beautiful tapestry to provide for all our needs.

A Tale of Two Parties

The day after my diagnosis—my thirty-fourth birthday—a friend picked me up and delivered me to a surprise party like no other. My arrival wasn't met with shouts of "Surprise!" but rather with lingering hugs from friends with tear-stained cheeks. Our toddlers played at our feet while we munched on snacks that had been hurriedly purchased the night before. I opened my gifts: stacks of paper plates to get my family through the difficult months to come and hand lotion to battle dry skin during chemotherapy. I had to step away from the party a few times in order to take phone calls from medical offices and to set up tests for the next day. And the party concluded with a lengthy time of weepy prayers as we pleaded with the Lord for comfort, peace, wisdom, and healing. Through the entire party, I kept wondering if I would live to see my thirty-fifth birthday. Would I be celebrating again with friends, or would it be a day of mourning as they marked my first birthday in heaven?

One year later, a crowd gathered on the lawn of a country house on a gorgeous October afternoon. Two of my childhood friends had flown in from Texas and California to throw me a thirty-fifth birthday party and celebrate my survival. There were only happy tears as guests filled their plates from a buffet of my favorite appetizers and desserts and listened to touching and humorous tributes. My denim skirt hung from my still-too-thin frame as everyone complimented the short, curly hair I had recently freed from underneath my wig. In my mind, my future was still uncertain. I expected a cancer recurrence at any time and didn't think I would live to see my fortieth birthday. But I was thankful for the Lord's healing. I was eager to give God the glory and praise for bringing me through the trial and preserving my life.

The battle of the previous year had been lengthy, painful, overwhelming, and emotional. And yet the Lord had proved faithful and present in each grueling step. My friends were there on the darkest days when I faced the reality of my prognosis and its implications for my young family. They were there on the days when I grasped at normalcy and wanted to be treated like a regular mom. They cried with me, prayed for me, and served my family tirelessly. I hope, as you read the stories throughout this book, you will feel equipped and inspired to love your friend through cancer as well as my friends loved me.

Questions for Reflection

1. Which of the "First Steps of Support," on the following page, could you take to help your friend today?
2. My friend said that God hadn't given the assignment of cancer to me as an individual—he had given this assignment to me and my community. What do you think about this statement?
3. God has given you specific gifts to be used to minister to your friend. What tangible, emotional, or spiritual resources has the Lord given you that you can share with her? You can write these down in Resource 1.1 (pg. 202).

FIRST STEPS OF SUPPORT

As you continue reading, here are some first steps you can take as you seek to respond to your friend's diagnosis with compassionate support:

☐ Pray for her. She needs your prayers more than anything—prayers for healing, strength, and support, for the ability to accept help, and for her relationship with the Lord. Chapter 10 provides specific ways to pray for your friend and specific Scriptures to use in your prayers.

☐ Offer to take her a meal (if she's an acquaintance) or set up an online meal calendar for her (if she's one of your closest friends).

☐ Drop off a large package of paper plates, breakfast or lunch items, or restaurant gift cards.

☐ Send a card in the mail letting her know you are praying for her.

☐ Don't assume that you know what she's feeling. Instead, ask questions and be prepared to listen well. You might want to skim chapter 4 to help you prepare for these conversations.

Circles

Knowing Your Role as a
Friend or Acquaintance

Our doorbell rang every Tuesday night at 5:30 for months. The young man at the door handed over a large half cheese, half pepperoni pizza without asking for payment. For the three young, picky eaters who lived under our roof, the weekly pizza delivery was a dream come true.

This kind gesture during my illness was arranged and paid for by a group of my husband's colleagues. To this day, I still don't know their names. They were not in our inner circle of friends. But they reached in from our outer circle of support and made a significant impact on our family's life for months.

If one of these men had offered to give me a ride to chemo, it would have felt awkward. I didn't want them to fold my laundry or clean my toilets. But they knew that as acquaintances, one of their primary roles was to provide food, and they did so with generosity and thoughtfulness.

Knowing where you fall in your friend's network of friends can help you determine the type of support to provide. She needs your support, regardless of whether you are in her inner circle of closest friends, a middle circle of friends and close acquaintances, or the outer circle of acquaintances. But the way you will support her should vary depending on how close your friendship is. Think of your friend as the center—the one who is experiencing the health crisis—and consider honestly where you stand in relation to her.

Determining Your Circle

In our social-media-obsessed culture, we often have a skewed perspective of the closeness of our friendships. Just because you know what your friend ate for dinner last night doesn't mean you are in her small circle of best friends. Take time to realistically consider where you fall within your friend's circles.

- How often do you communicate outside of social media?
- How often do you socialize?
- Do you share personal information with each other beyond superficial facts and opinions?
- Did she call you with the news of her diagnosis, or did you hear the news from others who are closer to her?

The inner circle includes her closest friends. Inner-circle friends talk, text, or visit frequently. Deeper discussions about your family, emotions, joys, and struggles form an essential aspect of your friendship. You know each other's loved ones well. You are familiar with each other's likes, dislikes, favorites, preferences, and personalities. When your basement floods, your baby won't sleep, or your teenager makes you crazy, you're in it together.

The middle circle includes friends with significant common interests. If you socialize occasionally, have more than a superficial relationship, or overlap in multiple spheres of life, you are probably in the middle circle. You may also be a middle-circle friend if you were in her inner circle in a previous season of life but don't communicate on a weekly basis anymore.

Middle-circle friends have a significant level of common interest or large areas of overlap in their lives. Maybe you've been in a small group together at church, your kids play together frequently in the neighborhood, or you enjoy a common hobby. You share personal information beyond what you would share with an acquaintance, but you probably aren't the first friend she would call in a crisis.

The outer circle includes acquaintances, online friends, and friends-of-friends who rally with support. If you know her well from one sphere of life but rarely socialize outside that sphere, you are probably an outer-circle friend. You chat after church on Sunday or at the gym. You keep in touch sporadically, but you don't see each other beyond that one place where your lives overlap. You may relate primarily using social media. You know where she took her last vacation, but you don't know her latest personal struggle.

To summarize, you can use this handy test to know your circle. Let's talk about your friend's dog for a minute:

- If you know from firsthand experience that your friend has a dog, the dog's name, and what the dog did last week to make your friend crazy, you're an inner-circle friend.
- If you know the dog's name and have met the dog, you're a middle-circle friend.
- If the only reason you know that your friend has a dog is because she posts about the dog on social media, you're an outer-circle friend.

If you've decided you're an outer-circle friend, don't put this book down! All the circles of friends have important roles to play. Remember our weekly pizza delivery? The population of someone's inner circle is small by nature, and the middle and outer circles are larger. It's likely that you will be in the middle or outer circles of most people who you know with cancer. But the support that you provide from those circles is valuable and critically important.

Once you've determined which circle most accurately describes your friendship, consider how your circle affects the support you should provide. Keep in mind that by showing up and supporting her consistently, you may find yourself moving inward among her circles of friends.

The Inner Circle

When you're thirty-four years old and are praying for your husband's next wife, you need a friend to share that pain with you. One early morning the week after my diagnosis, I sat curled up on my friend's sofa, dressed in sweatpants with my bare feet tucked underneath me. We wrapped our hands around mugs of hot coffee and cried. I told her I wanted my husband to remarry quickly if I died. I confessed that I had been praying for God to provide a second wife for him and a stepmom for my kids. I asked her to speak up and let others know my wishes, so that no one would resent my husband if he started dating.

Having these gut-wrenching conversations is one of the roles of an inner-circle friend. Your friend needs a safe place to wrestle through her difficult emotions. Other primary responsibilities of inner-circle friends include

- making sacrifices in order to serve your friend during this season of suffering
- giving emotional and spiritual support

- organizing the logistical support of other friends and acquaintances
- providing childcare (since her children probably feel comfortable with you)
- relaying information and support between your friend with cancer and her friends in the middle and outer circles
- protecting your friend and her family from gossip
- meeting other needs that require a close friend, such as accompanying her to medical appointments

When I was sick, my inner-circle friends sacrificed their own time, comfort, and convenience in order to serve me for several months. They cleaned my house, accompanied me to medical appointments, and even flew to Houston to care for me during chemotherapy treatments there. They organized several months of meals and made sure our logistical needs were covered. They served as a gate between the larger circles and me—protecting my time and my privacy while relaying information and needs to others.

My husband and I decided that our young children should be cared for by people they knew well in order to preserve stability for them. So this responsibility fell mainly to my inner-circle friends. They created an emotionally safe place for my kids during a remarkably unpredictable time in their lives. They took them on field trips and built gingerbread houses with them. And they sent me photos of my smiling children to encourage me when I couldn't be with them.

My inner circle also served as a safe place for my emotions. With courage and compassion, they walked with me though my dark days of struggling with the implications of my diagnosis. They spent time in understanding the details of the cancer I faced and my treatment plan. They knew the names of my doctors and when my next appointments were. One of my best friends even kept a spreadsheet of my platelet numbers for months, looking for trends and predicting when they would bottom out during each round of chemo. They were aware of how I was feeling on a daily basis—throughout almost a year of treatment and months into my survivorship. My inner-circle friends understand that today I still struggle with emotional implications of that phone call in 2010.

My closest friends could not do all this while also bringing me meals three times a week. And so my inner circle mobilized others in the outer circles to meet certain logistical needs. Because your friend probably doesn't want an acquaintance cleaning her bathroom or folding her underwear, some logistical tasks need to be done by an inner- or middle-circle friend. But those on the inside should delegate and communicate many of the logistical needs to the outer circles and should give them an opportunity to serve. Consider setting up a meal calendar or an online sign-up list to organize her needs. Your friend probably doesn't have the mental energy to devote to organizational tasks right now, and it will be difficult for her to know how to handle the onslaught of offers to help.

As an inner-circle friend, you will have information about your friend that is not meant for public knowledge. One of your roles is to protect your friend from gossip. She has a sensational, and potentially tragic, story. In our fallen nature, we are tempted to gossip about tragic stories. Resist the temptation to share information without your friend's permission. In situations when you are unsure of what to share, it's best to keep quiet or only share information that your friend has already shared publicly. If you hear others sharing gossip, step in and stand up for her.

Most importantly, ask your friend what she'd like you to say when people ask how she's doing. If she's struggling with how to respond, suggest a response and ask her what she thinks. For example, if she'd rather not share much information, suggest something simple: "Thank you for asking. She really would appreciate your prayers for her healing!" If she'd like to give a little more detail, suggest: "Thank you for asking. She starts treatment next month and would appreciate your prayers for complete restoration." But remember, as an inner-circle friend, you should have a response ready because you are sure to receive questions about your friend's condition. Knowing how you will respond will prevent you from being caught off guard, ensure that you honor your friend, and help you quell the rumor mill.

The Middle Circle

The text message was very specific: Callie, a young newlywed I had mentored the year before, let me know she had free time each morning before work. She asked if there were tasks she could cover on a regular basis—maybe she could drive one of my children to school?

This offer from a middle-circle friend met a huge need. One of my best friends (who had just had her fourth baby) was covering my share of our preschool carpool each week. So Callie began driving my son and my friend's daughter to preschool once a week, lessening the burden on my close friend and me.

Just as the circles of friends form concentric circles around the cancer patient, the responsibilities of the circles of friends also form concentric circles. Imagine the territory of the inner-circle friends as being the patient and the inside of her home: her emotions, her children, and her toilets. The realm of the middle circle is just beyond the home: the yard, transportation, errands, communicating support via mail or electronic communication, and popping into the home for short visits.

Here are the primary responsibilities of middle-circle friends:

- providing emotional support by checking in with your friend at least weekly
- assisting with logistical needs such as yard work, transportation, meals, and errands
- visiting her
- assisting inner-circle friends with logistical responsibilities of a personal nature, if needed

You should check in with your friend on a regular basis—every week or so—and set reminders if you won't remember on your own. But understand that you may not always hear back from her. Preface your messages by saying, "You don't have to write me back." Consistently and repeatedly let her know that you are thinking of her and care about her. Pray for your friend, let her know you are praying, and encourage her with promises from God's Word.

Appropriate logistical tasks for middle-circle friends include doing yard work, bringing meals, getting cars serviced, providing transportation to medical appointments, and running errands. Offer to pick up groceries when you're at the store, ask whether she needs anything from the pharmacy, or give her kids a ride to school or to extracurricular activities.

Chapter 7 includes a detailed list of logistical ways to serve your friend. Consider how you can serve her family, and make a specific offer of help. Depending on how private your friend is and how extensive her logistical needs are, you may or may not be called on for the inner-circle responsibilities.

Ask your friend if she'd enjoy visitors, but keep your visits short. Give her the opportunity to share how she's feeling about her diagnosis, and let her guide the conversation. Follow her lead if she changes the subject—she may not feel comfortable baring her soul to you just yet.

The Outer Circle

When I was sick, I loved getting notes in the mail. I received a note from the mother of our friend Jennifer, whose husband attended school with my husband. And then I started getting notes from the friends of Jennifer's mom. I've never met her, but she asked several people to pray for me and encourage me. I'm thankful for her willingness to reach out to a stranger with compassionate and sincere support. She is one example of the many outer-circle friends who intentionally showed their concern by sending me notes, prayers, and casseroles.

The outer circle includes acquaintances who rarely socialize outside of a common interest or who primarily interact online. As a member of the outer circle, you have these primary responsibilities:

- Bring food.
- Communicate support.
- Pray. Bring more food.

During my cancer treatment, my family received meals three times a week for eight months. That's over a hundred meals, and it wouldn't have happened without a large outer circle committed to feeding us! If your friend's treatment lasts several months, you may need to bring her multiple meals.

You should regularly communicate your support—even if it is just a short message that says, "I'm praying for you today!" Remember that cancer can be isolating, and she needs to hear constantly from her crowd of cheerleaders. When I posted updates on my CaringBridge website, I was so encouraged by the guest-book messages. Along with social media comments, these guest-book messages were easy ways for others to communicate their support without requiring a response from me.

Please don't stop praying for your friend. She needs your prayers for healing, strength, comfort, and peace. Consider organizing a prayer meeting and join with others to pray. Text or email your prayers to your friend. Add her name to the intercessory prayer list at your church. If she posts public social media updates, share them with others and ask for their prayers. Then let her know of your constant, continued prayers. I cherished every note I received that let me know someone was praying for me. (See chapter 10 for specific ways you can lift up your friend in prayer.)

Outer-circle friends can also rally to meet financial needs caused by your friend's medical expenses or time away from work. A large network of supporters who each have a little to give can significantly ease your friend's financial burdens. Be aware of fundraising efforts, and show your support by contributing if you are able. You might consider organizing others to give, whether through an online effort, a live event, or the sale of T-shirts or other products to raise money for her medical bills.

You might also look for ways to support inner-circle friends who are making frequent sacrifices in order to serve your friend. On occasion, a mutual friend provided a meal for my friend as she spent time caring for my children. It was a beautiful example of the body of Christ working together.

Remember, these guidelines are meant to be helpful ideas, not hard-and-fast rules. Use prayerful discernment to know how God is calling you to serve and support your friend. Ask your friend directly, or those in her inner circle, how you can serve most helpfully.

Questions for Reflection

1. What is your perception of your friend's support network and where you stand in it?
2. Are your friend's logistical needs extensive, typical, or minimal? Will she need a larger circle of friends sharing the burden, or can it be handled by a few close friends? How does this affect what your role will be?
3. Which of the responsibilities listed for your circle resonate most with you? Are there responsibilities outside your circle that you feel called to fulfill as well?

ACTION STEPS TO CONSIDER

All friends:

☐ Consider realistically where you fall in her circle of friends.

☐ Use the examples given in this chapter to prayerfully consider how you can help with your friend's unique needs.

☐ Avoid the urge to gossip or share what you know about your friend's condition (unless she's given you permission to share).

☐ Set a weekly alarm or calendar entry to remind you to communicate your love and support through a text, email, or phone call.

☐ Keep gently pursuing your friend, even if she doesn't respond.

☐ Read Resource 2.1: A Biblical View of Community for a better understanding of the importance of the community surrounding your friend.

☐ If both you and she are married, go a step further and hand your husband Resource 2.2: A Letter to Your Husband about Her Husband, so that your family can get involved in supporting her family as well.

Inner-circle friends:

☐ Listen and provide encouragement as she grapples with difficult emotions.

☐ Ease the burden on your friend by serving as a point person to relay updates and needs to the middle and outer circles.

- [ ] Care for her children, provide stability and fun, and be aware of their emotional needs.

- [ ] Assist with logistical tasks that are private in nature, such as accompanying her to medical appointments.

Middle-circle friends:
- [ ] Check in frequently with your friend to communicate support without expecting a response.

- [ ] Perform tasks that are essential but slightly less personal, such as yard work, transportation, or running errands.

- [ ] Visit her, but keep it short.

Outer-circle friends:
- [ ] Communicate support in ways that don't necessitate a response.

- [ ] Bring food, and do so repeatedly if her treatment is lengthy.

- [ ] Pray without ceasing.

- [ ] Participate in fundraising efforts.

- [ ] Support those in the inner and middle circles.

When the Going Gets Tough

Struggles You Will Face

When my friend Sarah's close friend was diagnosed with cancer, their circle of friends seemed to grow overnight. At first the new faces felt threatening. Sarah wanted to serve her friend and take care of her, and she wondered, *What are all these other people doing here?* Sometimes she felt insecure as she watched other friends serve in ways that she hadn't thought of. Janet faced the opposite problem when her best friend battled metastatic breast cancer. She watched friends walk away when they couldn't handle the situation, and it broke Janet's heart.

It's difficult having a friend with cancer. You probably felt shocked, scared, and sad when you heard your friend's diagnosis. You hate seeing her endure pain, weakness, nausea, and other side effects of treatment. Even though you're not enduring the same physical suffering that your friend is, you are still suffering with her. In Resource 3.1 we will dive deeper into the issue of suffering, so I recommend reading it when you're ready.

This chapter will discuss the struggles you will face as you watch your friend suffer. I encountered many of these firsthand when I walked with family members and friends through cancer. I don't want you to be caught off guard if you encounter them too. Even if there aren't easy solutions, sometimes it's comforting to know that you're not the only one who has felt the way you feel.

You May Feel Threatened by Her Other Friendships

Over time, Sarah learned that God had grown her friend's circle because her friend needed an army of helpers. Caring for a friend through months of chemotherapy is a marathon. Along the way, friends will have their own crises to deal with and will need to step back from helping. Or they may grow weary and need another friend to step in for a while. Overwhelming logistical needs are better handled by a large group of committed friends.

Now Sarah's advice to friends of cancer patients is to welcome the new faces. Get to know the additions to your friend's circle. You'll be working together for months, and possibly years, to support your mutual friend. Don't set a precedent of doing it all yourself. If you do, the others might leave, thinking that you've got it all under control, and then you'll find yourself needing them. Besides, these new faces will probably become your friends, too. Don't push them away. You need each other and might find yourself enjoying these new friendships.

You May Wear Yourself Out

Sarah also felt a strong drive to do everything for her friend. She was hurting and sad about her friend's diagnosis, and serving her friend helped her feel a bit better. But she quickly learned to stop thinking she could love her friend the best by serving her the most. If you try to be the superhero, you'll find yourself burned out and exhausted before your friend is finished needing you.

Letting others enter the inner circle and have an opportunity to serve is one solution to the caregiver burnout problem. Another solution is to establish healthy boundaries.

I'm guessing that you didn't have a lot of free time before your friend was diagnosed with cancer, right? You weren't sitting around looking for ways to fill your time? In fact, you were probably overwhelmed already by the demands of family, work, and daily tasks. Most of us operate without much margin in our schedule—I know I do! And now your friend needs you. She needs meals. She needs rides. She needs your listening ear. She needs you to help with her kids. You may be wondering, *How in the world am I going to pull this off?*

You need to understand something very important: You are absolutely not going to do all these things for your friend. You are one link in her support chain. You'll have ways in which you are specifically called and gifted to support her, and other friends will be called and gifted to support her in different ways.

A few years ago, a woman in my Bible study shared that she needed a biopsy the following week. She'd had an abnormal mammogram, and the biopsy was the next step. She needed someone to drive her to the appointment, and I assumed that it should be me. Who better to take her and be with her if the worst happened? Of course it should be me!

But there was a problem. Her appointment was on a day when I was homeschooling my children. I tried unsuccessfully to find a babysitter. I slowly started to realize that I was going to have to tell my friend I couldn't take her. I dreaded making that phone call. I put it off as long as possible, not wanting to let her down and worrying about what she would think of me. But when I had exhausted all of my childcare options, I knew I had to make the call. I dialed her number and hoped for her voicemail. When she answered and I apologetically explained that I couldn't take her, she replied, "Oh! That's okay! Suzie already said she could take me!"

I've seen this happen over and over again. Many times I knew that a friend with cancer had a need—a legitimate, important need—that I could not meet. I racked my brain, trying to figure out a way to take care of it, when I knew deep down that God wasn't asking me to do it. And, every single time, I saw God bring along someone else who was able to meet that need. It was never my job in the first place! In my pride, I often forget that God is using the entire body of Christ to provide for my friends. When we place our friend's needs in the Lord's hands, we are free to serve without the pressure to do it all.

You May Struggle to Find Balance

When Sarah served her friend with cancer, she realized how important it was to care for her own family first. When her responsibilities were taken care of, she could serve her friend from a place of freedom. She needed to communicate clearly with her friend how she could serve and also make sure that her friend knew when she wasn't available to help. This can be challenging when the schedule of a cancer patient is unpredictable! There are times when you'll need to stick to your schedule and other times when you'll need to be flexible. Just keep praying and communicating, and trust God with the details.

If you're a close friend, you may be constantly aware of her needs. And you might feel tempted to jump in and offer to help without being asked. In fact, this is one of my tips in later chapters—anticipating your friend's needs is one great way to serve her. But be careful. Don't always jump in without being asked. Step back, let your friend float the request to her team of supporters, and see if someone else feels called to meet that need.

As you walk through this with your friend, please protect

yourself and your family by setting boundaries on your time and energy. Pray about how God is asking you to serve her. Ask him if there are responsibilities you need to put on hold while you serve your friend, while realizing that you can't put your entire life on hold indefinitely. If you're married, ask your husband how much time he thinks you can commit to serving your friend. Prayerfully decide how you can serve, and stick with your decision. Then trust God to meet your friend's needs.

You May Feel Guilty Enjoying Your Life

When my sister-in-law battled cancer the year before I did, her first round of chemo fell during when our family's vacation had been planned. The dates had been set long before we knew of her diagnosis, and she didn't need our help during that round, so we continued on with our plans. But I felt terrible for enjoying a vacation while she was suffering. I felt like an awful friend as I laughed and played with my family at a water park while knowing that she planned to shave her head. She was never far from my thoughts that week.

Even today, when I visit a friend at chemo, it feels bizarre to leave the oncology clinic and go pick up groceries or have a date night with my husband. It feels selfish. Sometimes I don't even want my friend to know that I'm out doing normal things while she's home in bed.

But here's the truth: You need to live the life God has given you right now. Your friend needs to live the life he has given her. You aren't doing her any good by feeling guilty about the circumstances the Lord has sovereignly ordained for you. There will be days when you're immersed in the pain your friend is feeling, walking alongside her in her suffering. Your world will revolve around her some of the time. But you also need to spend time enjoying your health and joyful circumstances.

That is okay to do. It's more than okay—it is wonderful to enjoy the gifts that God gives you!

Try not to live inside your friend's head or imagine what she must feel like. Sympathize, yes. But you can't truly empathize with her or imagine what she feels like unless you yourself have had cancer—and, even then, you haven't been in her specific circumstances with her unique personality and response to suffering, so you aren't equipped to accurately imagine her unique grief, devastation, and fears.

God is pouring out grace to meet her needs, like the manna he sent to the Israelites in the desert. She is receiving the cancer manna. The Lord will daily provide the strength that she needs to face her circumstances. God's provision for her doesn't take her pain away, but he will be faithful to sustain her through this difficulty, one day at a time. You don't have cancer, so you're not receiving the cancer manna. You're receiving the Lord's provision for your situation—the cancer-friend manna. He is with you, and he will sustain you as well. But the grace you're receiving is different from the grace the Lord is pouring out on your friend.

If you try to take on your friend's thoughts and feelings, they will crush you. The cancer-friend manna doesn't provide what you need in order to live as though cancer is happening to you. Don't constantly put yourself in her emotional shoes without the grace that God is giving her to walk in those shoes. It will lead to despair. Live the life that God is giving you.

You May Miss the Old Days

Your friendship will be different from now on. It's a hard reality, but it's true. During your friend's physical battle, you need to let your friendship be one-sided, not expecting to receive anything from her. It's all giving on your part. And, when her treatment ends, you'll probably notice that your friend has changed, and therefore your friendship may feel different. You may experience a sense of loss as you grieve the friendship you were accustomed to.

When Lisa's friend endured months of chemo, Lisa missed spending time with her. Her heart broke each time that she picked up her friend's kids for school events. She wished she were meeting her friend there and chatting about their week like they used to. Lisa felt guilty watching her friend stay home while she went about her normal life, and she missed her friend.

It's tough being in a one-sided friendship. Your friend needs you to provide support to her, and she won't have much to give you in return. You don't need to remain emotionless in front of her, but don't expect her to comfort you about her cancer. I understand that you need comfort—this is so hard. Please find a trustworthy friend or counselor to talk with about your struggles and emotions. You need a place to vent, but don't vent to your friend with cancer. Look for someone in her circles of friends who is further removed from your friend than you are, and ask for support from her.

Let yourself grieve the loss of your old friendship. I know it was hard on my friends when I had cancer, because they missed me. Instead of going to Bible study with me, they were juggling extra kids as they took mine along. We didn't grab lunch together or have girls' night out. I didn't offer to keep their kids while they went to the dentist or got their hair cut. And when you're the mom of littles, you need all hands on deck. It's difficult to lose a team member!

You May Fear Losing Her

You may also be afraid that your friend might die. Maybe she's facing a poor prognosis and is unlikely to survive. Or maybe you're bracing yourself for the unexpected turns that cancer sometimes brings.

When Jill Lynn Buteyn's friend Kara entered hospice care, Jill Lynn wrote these words:

> The idea that one day she won't be here to answer a text or dream big with me is . . . unfathomable. I'm supposed to be mourning her. But how do you mourn someone who's still alive? . . .
>
> I don't know how to let Kara go.
>
> And truthfully I'm not supposed to yet. She's still here. . . .
>
> How do you live while your friend is dying?
>
> You go on loving your family. You hug your husband. You still laugh. You catch yourself, wonder if you should be laughing, and then laugh some more. Because yes, we all have to keep living.[1]

I can relate. I've lost friends to cancer, and I'm terrified of losing more. I've wept as I tucked in my children at night and thought about my friend's children. I've struggled to find words of comfort or hope when my friend said, "I don't know how to do this. I don't know how to face the end."

When Janet's friend faced terminal cancer, she was convinced that her friend would beat it. Janet never let herself think about her friend dying. One day, her friend said they needed to talk about when she was gone. Janet said she couldn't talk about that yet, and they never returned to the conversation. Now that her friend has passed away, Janet wonders what her friend wanted to say. She wishes she would have been willing to have the discussion when her friend brought it up, or at least to come back to it quickly.

Janet sought counsel from a chaplain as her friend neared the end. Janet had no idea how to walk that road with her friend. The chaplain told her, "God will lead you." As difficult as the situation proved to be, Janet found the chaplain's words to be true. God was with them every step of the way.

I don't have an easy answer for you as you struggle with your friend's mortality. But remember the manna principle: God will give you what you need when you need it. If your friend isn't dying today, it's hard to imagine how you will ever face the heartbreak of losing her. Cling to the knowledge that, when the day comes, God will meet you there. He will give you the grace to endure. In the meantime, acknowledge that it's hard. Find a safe person to process your feelings with (though, again, this shouldn't be your friend with cancer). Let yourself grieve. Run with your sorrow into the arms of your heavenly Father and remember that nothing can separate you from his love (see Rom. 8:38–39).

As you struggle with your role as the friend of a cancer-fighter, you are not alone. I hope that by highlighting these challenges you may face, I've encouraged you to be honest with yourself and others about your struggles. Yes, it is hard. But there will also be joy. Lisa has struggled with balancing her friend's needs and her own family's needs, and she has grieved the loss of their pre-cancer friendship. But she also sees the spiritual fruit that has grown in her family as they've served their friends and watched the Lord work in their trial. One of my closest friends says that my cancer was a turning point in her walk with the Lord, deepening her trust and dependence on him.

I hope you will also see how God is at work in you and your family through your involvement in your friend's suffering. Ask a trusted friend or a pastor to guide and encourage you as you wrestle with your own emotions surrounding your friend's illness, welcoming new friends, balancing your desire to serve with your own needs, feeling guilty about your health, missing your friendship, and fearing your friend's death. Cry out to the Lord with your worries and fears. And walk confidently alongside your friend, trusting the Lord to provide exactly what both of you need.

Questions for Reflection

1. What are your previous experiences with cancer? What baggage are you carrying into your friend's journey?
2. Which of the struggles outlined in this chapter do you think will be difficult for you?
3. Who can you process these struggles with? (This should be someone who is further removed than you are from your friend with cancer—who is more outside in her circle of friends.)

ACTION STEPS TO CONSIDER

☐ Talk through your emotions regarding your friend's diagnosis with a trusted pastor, counselor, or friend who is further removed from the situation.

☐ Welcome your friend's new friends into her circle of support.

☐ Don't try to meet all your friend's needs on your own. Set healthy boundaries, pray for wisdom, and trust God to provide for her.

☐ Care for your own family first, and then consider how you can serve your friend. Give others the opportunity to jump in and help.

☐ Don't feel guilty enjoying your healthy life—live freely in the circumstances the Lord has given you.

☐ Let yourself grieve the loss of the way your friendship used to be, and run to the Lord with your fears for your friend's future.

☐ Read Resource 3.1: A Biblical View of Suffering to gain understanding and encouragement as you suffer alongside your friend.

When Religious Platitudes Fail You

How to Avoid Saying the Wrong Thing

Have you ever dodged a friend or acquaintance who was going through something difficult because you didn't know what to say? I have. Our fear of not finding the right words to encourage or comfort often holds us back from providing the support our friends need. I hate to tell you this, but our fears are not unfounded. Every cancer survivor or caregiver I've spoken with has stories of friends who hurt their feelings with well-intentioned remarks.

Jennifer was forced to listen to her daughter's teacher describe the painful impact of her mother's death from cancer when she was a child. As a mom of school-aged kids and a metastatic cancer patient, this was the last thing Jennifer needed to hear. The teacher started the conversation by saying that Jennifer was in her thoughts and prayers. She should have stopped right there.

I know that many of us know better than this teacher—we would never share a horror story that would upset our friends. But I'm probably not the only one who has said the wrong thing and wished I could take it back. I'm not the only one who's been afraid to reach out with support because I might say the wrong thing. If you share these fears, keep reading. In this chapter, we will explore several ways to avoid saying the wrong thing to your friend with cancer. We'll learn how to say less, choose questions carefully, skip religious platitudes, and think about the impact of our words and whether they'll communicate the support we are eager to give.

Just Say Less

Here's one guaranteed way not to say the wrong thing: say nothing at all. Proverbs 10:19 teaches us that "when words are many, transgression is not lacking, but whoever restrains his lips is prudent." This is the perfect guiding principle for our interactions with friends with cancer. Say less; listen more. If your friend doesn't have anything to say, sit with her in silence.

Dietrich Bonhoeffer writes,

> Christians, especially ministers, so often think they must always contribute something when they are in the company of others, that this is the one service they have to render. They forget that listening can be a greater service than speaking.
>
> Many people are looking for an ear that will listen. They do not find it among Christians, because these Christians are talking where they should be listening.[1]

Although these words were written decades ago, it's as if Bonhoeffer were a fly on the wall of twenty-first-century coffee shops, homes, and hospital rooms. We head into our interactions with hurting people thinking about the reassurance we can offer them. We've got our Bibles, we've rehearsed prayers that sound like sermons, and we're ready to speak words of hope. Our Bibles, prayers, and hopeful words have their place. But first comes listening and silence.

Kara Tippetts, a young mom and wife, wrote these words during her battle with terminal breast cancer: "There is so much power in showing up, humble power in saying, 'I'm here. I may not have the answers, but I'm here.' Most often it's those who come without answers or agendas who are the most helpful."[2]

Jess, whose infant daughter battled neuroblastoma, told me how much she appreciated friends who were willing to sit with them in silence. She said, "Their presence is even more important than what they say. People surrounding you, even if they don't say anything, means a lot."

Not saying much is hard. We want to help our friend move past her pain and feel better. We want this because we love our friend, and we don't want her to hurt anymore. We also want this because her pain makes us uncomfortable. We're eager to move past her pain into safer territory.

But, if we are going to love our friend well, it's imperative that we sit with her in the pit of her hard emotions. Don't offer a ladder out of the pit that won't feel real to your friend. Don't let her see you looking around for a way out because you're uncomfortable. Just sit with her. Cry with her. Be silent with her. The ministry of silence will not be easy for you, but it will be comforting to your friend.

Be Careful with Your Questions

One of the most frequent questions I heard when I had cancer was, "How did you discover the cancer? Did you find a lump?" This isn't a bad question, but it didn't make me feel supported. Questions like these demonstrate curiosity, not concern. The question has nothing to do with how I'm feeling today, what I need, or how you can support me. It arises from your need to feel better about your own health, and it asks me to put your mind at ease about how you can avoid a similar situation.

Part of listening to your friend involves asking good questions, but you must be careful with the questions you ask. Here are three questions to ask yourself before you ask your friend a question.

1. Am I curious or caring?

In *Just Show Up*, Jill Buteyn writes, "Curiosity is different from caring. . . . Curiosity wants to know what's going on. Caring wants the person to know they're not forgotten. Details aren't important."[3]

Curiosity asks,

- How much longer do you have to live?
- Will you need a mastectomy?
- Are you getting a second opinion?
- Did you have genetic testing?
- What are the chances of recurrence?

Caring asks,

- Are you feeling hopeful or discouraged today?
- How are you feeling about the physical implications of your treatment?
- Do you have appointments coming up this week that I can pray for?
- How are you processing this diagnosis with your family members?
- Do you have fears you need to talk about?

I love information. I crave details. I want to know everything that is going on in my friend's mind, especially when she's going through something as significant as cancer. Sometimes, when I ask questions that may come across as curious, I'm truly motivated by concern. But often my questions are motivated by a desire for information in order to put my own mind at ease. If you're a close friend, I know that it's difficult to walk alongside your friend without knowing all the details. But you can love her well by putting your needs aside and being content with the information she gives. Your friend will feel supported by questions that flow from caring, not curiosity.

2. Am I trying to fix a problem or understand a person?

Imagine pouring out your heart about a deep concern, only to have your listener go straight into fix-it mode without trying to understand your emotions and needs. I won't forget the person who responded to my cancer story with "Did you ever consider alternative medicine?"

Our drive to fix problems is powerful. We want to offer advice, make sure our friend has all the available options, and be the hero who makes the winning suggestion—whether we're tackling emotional, medical, spiritual, or logistical issues. But your friend doesn't need fixing; she needs understanding.

When we try to fix, we make it about us. Our information, our suggestions, our wisdom, our solutions. When we seek to understand, we make it about our friend. Her sadness, her struggles, her challenges. Before you ask a question, check your motives. Are you trying to be a hero or a hearer?

3. Am I close enough to ask this question?

If you've been pregnant, you've probably experienced the phenomenon of complete strangers asking personal questions. They ask when you're due. They ask what you're having and whether it's your first. They may even want to touch your belly.

The same is true of a cancer patient—especially if she is a woman with breast cancer. Why do people think that, all of a sudden, it's okay to talk about our breasts? Here's the thing: it's not okay. It's personal and probably emotional, and this territory needs to be treaded carefully.

Some cancer patients are open about their health and treatment. Your friend may talk freely about her surgical options and their implications. In the months during and after my treatment, I joked that at any given time there was an 80 percent chance that I was talking to someone about my chest. But others may not feel comfortable sharing this information outside of a very small circle of friends and family.

Here's a good rule of thumb to remember: A topic that you regularly discussed with your friend before she had cancer is probably safe now. If you never in a million years would have asked your friend if her breasts were fake before cancer, it's not appropriate to ask today. If you used to talk about marital struggles, it's okay to ask how her spouse is handling her diagnosis. If your conversations before cancer centered around the weather, stick with asking her how she feels about the recent drop in temperatures and wait to see if she brings up more intimate topics.

Skip the Religious Platitudes

When I talk to cancer-fighters and caregivers, there is one theme that emerges when I ask, "What did people say or do that wasn't helpful?" Over and over again, I hear that the least helpful comments are religious platitudes such as "God is in control," "God has a plan," and "God works all things for good." If you're anything like me, that sentence probably made you uncomfortable. On the inside, you're shouting at me, "But it's true! God is in control! He has a plan! He works all things together for good!" Yes, I know. I'm shouting at myself in my head, too. I've gotten this wrong repeatedly when walking with friends through suffering. I've had to apologize and ask for forgiveness. It's taken me years to learn that these statements, while true and biblical, are usually not comforting or helpful when a sister in Christ is hurting.

The most common response heard by suffering people is something along the lines of "All things work out for good in the end." This is true. It is straight out of the Bible—in fact, it is one of my favorite verses. Romans 8:28 says, "And we know that for those who love God all things work together for good, for those who are called according to his purpose." Romans 8:28 is true. Romans 8:28 is good. But, when your friend is suffering, it is not the time for Romans 8:28. At that moment, Romans 8:28 will feel like a fake "happy Jesus stamp" placed on something that feels difficult, sad, and scary for your friend. It may cause your friend to feel that you don't understand her, that you are flippant with her trauma, or that you are not a safe place when she is struggling.

As I've talked about this with believers who have suffered and heard these words, I've noticed three reasons why Romans 8:28 and other religious platitudes aren't just unhelpful but can actually damage our relationship with the hurting friend and our attempts to comfort her.

1. Your friend will think you think that she doesn't know this.

If your friend affirms God's sovereignty, the implication that she doesn't will feel insulting. And the last thing she needs to feel right now is insulted. If your friend doesn't believe God's sovereignty, then the words will be meaningless to her. Either way, your words will fail to bring comfort to your friend.

Many of my friends who have walked this road told me

that when people said these things, it hurt because it implied that the suffering person didn't already know it. What they heard was, "Clearly you've forgotten that God is in charge. Your tears and grief tell me that you aren't trusting the good Lord's good plans for you."

My friends knew the truth about the Lord. They believed it with all their hearts. But they were still sad, still hurting, still afraid, and still wishing that God's plans were different. They didn't need a Bible teacher. They needed someone to sit with them in their pain and cry with them.

What if your friend isn't a Christian, or if she struggles with doubt to the extent that she doesn't believe God's Word is true? This is a tough situation. In Resource 2.1, we discuss how Scripture exhorts us to serve our friends who don't believe as we do. Our discussion throughout this book focuses primarily on how to encourage our Christian friends, and we will need to use wisdom when applying these principles to those who aren't walking with the Lord.

My friend Marilyn lost her father to cancer when she was twenty-two years old. She was a Christian, but her knowledge and belief had not yet transformed into a deep, abiding trust in the Lord. She spent years reeling from the loss of her dad. Life was hard. Suddenly, she was responsible for paying her way through a college career that had been put on hold when her dad got sick and finances became tight. It felt unfair to her that she had to face this trial when other people her age weren't losing their parents.

Marilyn's friends didn't get it. They didn't understand her loss or the pain that accompanied it, so she heard a lot of clichés and religious platitudes. And not one of them helped her to trust the Lord more deeply—they simply made her mad. They made her feel isolated and misunderstood.

Thirteen years later, Marilyn started attending a Bible

study that walked verse-by-verse through the Bible. Although she never walked away from her faith, she hadn't studied God's Word that way before. God used that Bible study to finally give her peace about her father's death. She is now convinced of the truth of God's promises—not only as head knowledge but as heartfelt rest. She has faced other hardships since and has seen the difference that these truths make in her response. She sees God's good timing in the struggles of her twenties and how he brought her to this place.

Marilyn's story inspires me to trust God when a friend struggles with doubt or unbelief. We need to be open to the Lord's guidance and speak truth when he calls us to. But when he calls us to comfort, we can do just that. We can leave the correction to him and his timing. We can trust him to use all things for our friend's good—even her struggles to believe.

2. It will feel like you're dismissing her pain or wanting her to hurry up her grief.

When Alexis's mom battled breast cancer, she felt rushed in her grief by friends who spoke in platitudes. She needed her friends to be okay with her sadness. She told me, "When someone says, 'God has a plan,' it feels like they're saying, 'Hurry up and be okay.'"

We desperately want to fix our friend's sadness, fear, or anger. This drive to fix is so deeply ingrained that we often don't realize how powerful a motivator it is. We are uncomfortable with difficult emotions. We want our friend to feel better, because we love her so deeply. We think that if we can correct her thinking, we can take away some of her pain. But we're wrong. Cancer is painful no matter how convinced you are of God's sovereignty.

We also want to ease our own discomfort in the midst of her grief. We don't know what to say. We don't know what to do. If we're honest, part of our motivation in using these words is to move the situation into more comfortable territory for our sake.

The truth of God's character keeps us from being crushed by our circumstances, but it doesn't take away our pain and sadness. When we understand this truth about suffering, we give our friend the freedom to take the time she needs with her emotions. We won't rush her. We won't try to correct her doctrine in an attempt to move her from sadness to joy in the midst of heartbreaking circumstances.

3. It will not accomplish your goal of communicating compassionate support to your friend.

Let's step back and think about your goal for your conversation with your friend. Is your goal to teach or correct doctrine? Is your goal to preach to her? Or is your goal to comfort her? To show your support and love for her? Do you want her to walk away feeling rebuked, corrected, and misunderstood? Or do you want her to feel heard, seen, and loved?

I love God's Word. I love the truth of the promises, doctrine, history, narratives, poetry, laments, and wisdom it contains. I affirm its inerrancy, relevancy, and goodness. But different passages are appropriate at different times. For example, I've never heard a pastor lead into a baptism by reading the story in Genesis 20 of Abraham pretending that Sarah was his sister and giving her to the king as a wife. The story is true, but its purpose doesn't fit with the occasion.

If our purpose is to show empathy and support, then we should use words and Scripture that fit with our purpose. Remember, every single cancer-fighter and caregiver I've talked with has told me that platitudes such as "God has a plan," "God is sovereign," and "God will use this for good" don't make them feel understood or loved. They don't bring comfort to their hurting souls. These phrases feel like a Bible verse Band-Aid slapped on their raw wounds.

In my experience, verses reminding us of God's presence with us are comforting and reassuring. Look for psalms that speak of God as our refuge and strength, such as Psalm 46. Encourage your friend with Scriptures that convey God's peace, comfort, help, and faithfulness. You'll find a great list in Resource 4.1 to get you started.

Let's use words and Scripture that are a balm to our friends' souls. Let's use our words to show that we understand their heartbreak and pain, not to diminish it. Let's tell our friends with cancer that we're sorry for their suffering, we love them, and we support them.

Don't Make It about You

Often when we say the wrong thing, it's because we're talking about ourselves or relating our friends' experience to ourselves rather than focusing on their pain. Here are some examples.

"I know how you feel . . . I was really sick when I was pregnant / had the stomach flu / etc."

Confession time: When my sister-in-law went through chemo the year before I did, I spent months comparing her chemo-related nausea to my pregnancy-related nausea. I still can't believe she didn't hang up on me every time. I was trying to empathize and find a shared experience in order to commiserate with her. What I didn't realize is that chemo nausea and pregnancy nausea have very little in common. Pregnancy and the stomach bug can make you feel terrible, but they do not carry all the emotional implications that come with cancer and chemotherapy. The experiences may all include vomiting, but they are worlds apart. Just don't go there. Instead, offer to bring her a smoothie or milkshake if it sounds good to her queasy stomach.

"I've always wanted a boob job! I'm so jealous!"

We'll talk more about mastectomies and breast reconstruction in chapter 6. But since this topic can often lead to verbal missteps, it's worth mentioning here as well. Please remember that if your friend needs breast reconstruction due to cancer, she is not getting a boob job. No matter how bravely or humorously your friend discusses her visits to the plastic surgeon, losing one or both breasts is excruciatingly difficult—physically and emotionally. She'll probably endure multiple surgeries, and she may or may not be pleased with the results. Even if she's happier than she expected to be, she will still look different than she did before cancer, and she will need to grieve the loss of her pre-cancer body. Remember, she didn't choose to have this surgery!

Don't joke about your friend's plastic surgery. (But do laugh if she jokes about it!) Don't tell her how jealous you are—trust me, she is jealous of your natural, imperfect, healthy breasts. And if you've had cosmetic breast surgery, she may not want to hear the details, and she definitely doesn't want you to compare your experience to hers. Instead, ask how she's coping with the changes to her body and how you can support her.

"I'm really upset this is happening to you. I hardly slept at all last night because I'm so worried!"

I don't want to be harsh, because I know that your friend's diagnosis is difficult for you. We hate to see our friends suffer. If a close friend's child has cancer, we may watch our own children struggle through their concern for their friend, and the emotions are intense. But it's important to not ask your friend to comfort you.

When Pam's three-year-old son battled cancer, one of her friends talked about how hard the situation was for her daughter, because the children were close friends. Pam didn't need the additional burden of hearing how her life-altering event was difficult for others. She needed their support, not the other way around. Aimee had a similar experience when her son battled cancer. She didn't want to have to comfort others, and she didn't want her teenage son to see others crying because of his illness.

I know that you're upset and worried and scared and sad. Having a friend with cancer is horribly difficult—trust me, I know. As we discussed in chapter 3, you need to have a friend who can help you work through these emotions. And your friend with cancer will not be that person. When you are with your friend, be concerned only about her emotions. It's okay to let her see that you are upset—it lets her know that you care. But don't expect her to support or comfort you. This friendship is going to be one-sided for a while, and you are the giving side. (The article "How Not to Say the Wrong Thing" listed in the For Further Reading section is a great resource for understanding more about this.)

"I read this article last night about a cancer-fighting diet/food/supplement/etc."

Your friend has an oncologist, right? In fact, she probably has an entire medical team. When I had cancer, I had so many doctors that I could hardly remember all their names. Your friend may be overwhelmed already by the information that her doctors are giving her. She doesn't need medical advice from anyone else. Let her doctors be the doctors. They went to school for a dozen years for this purpose.

Do you know why the internet overflows with articles about cancer-fighting [fill-in-the-blank]? Because people are terrified of cancer. Articles about cancer-fighting whatevers receive a multitude of likes and shares on social media. But many of those articles aren't founded on real science. Your friend's doctors are reading scientific studies written by other doctors about how to fight this cancer. Leave the job to them.

At this point, you may be upset with me if you're eager to share valid, useful information with your friend. If so, I'll make a compromise with you. You may send one email to your friend letting her know that you've done research (or have walked this road yourself) and that you have information that may be helpful to her. Let her know you'd be happy to share the information if she's interested. Then wait to see if she asks before you share more.

Rather than jumping in to offer advice, you should take the time to find out the details of your friend's medical treatment. Understand the terminology, treatment plan, and possible side effects. Depending on how openly she discusses these topics, this information may come from your friend or from reputable websites.

Other True (but Unhelpful) Statements to Avoid

Here are just a few more things to avoid saying when talking to your friend with cancer. These statements are unhelpful, discouraging, or minimizing to your friend's painful experience.

"It's just hair. It will grow back!"

Can you imagine the trauma of watching all the hair on your head gradually falling out? Waking up to clumps of hair on your pillow? Having it come out by the fistful in the shower?

68

All while receiving harsh treatment for a life-threatening disease? Unless you've experienced any of these firsthand, you can't truly imagine it. Yes, it's just hair. And yes, it will grow back. But, depending on how long her chemo lasts, she will be bald for several months. She may lose her eyelashes and eyebrows. If she braves public without a wig, she will receive stares of shock and pity. People may mistake her for a man. When her hair grows back, it will probably take years for it to resemble her pre-cancer hairstyle. Her baldness, and then her super-short hair, will be a constant reminder of the unwanted change to her life and her health.

Your friend knows that her hair loss is a cosmetic concern. She may even feel guilt over how devastated she feels to lose it. She needs your sympathy and understanding. Instead of minimizing her pain, ask how she's feeling. Offer to shop with her for a wig or pretty scarves. We'll talk more about hair loss and how to provide support through it in chapter 6.

"My great-aunt/neighbor/etc. had that cancer a few years ago. It didn't turn out well."

I understand that you are trying to relate to your friend and share her experience when you say this. Many of us have emotional baggage related to cancer, and those experiences may come to mind when we are talking to our friends. But please be careful when sharing stories about someone you know, whether they had cancer in general or had the same type of cancer that your friend has.

If your friend has just been diagnosed with breast cancer, she doesn't want to hear about people you know who died of colon cancer. It's upsetting and discouraging. She probably doesn't even want to hear about people you know who survived colon cancer—it's irrelevant to her. She *definitely* doesn't want to hear about people you know who died of breast cancer.

It may be helpful to share stories of people you know who have survived breast cancer, especially if those ladies are willing to reach out and offer support after their experience. But keep in mind that even within one type of cancer, such as breast cancer, there are many different sub-types and countless variations between cases and treatment plans. If you know someone who might be a good contact for your friend, throw the idea out there, but let your friend take the lead. She might not be ready yet.

There is one exception. If your friend has a rare cancer, it may be appropriate for you to share the story of someone else who had that specific cancer if it could provide useful or encouraging medical information. For example, if you know someone who is diagnosed with angiosarcoma, please tell her my story. Those of us with rare cancers need to stick together!

"Studies show that cancer patients with a positive attitude are more likely to survive. You just need to believe that you're going to beat this!"

I heard this and read this often when I had cancer. I haven't read the studies, so I can't say it's not true. I think it's good to be optimistic and hopeful. I think cancer patients should focus on having a fighting attitude, at least as long as the doctors offer hope of treatment. I also believe that God is sovereign over every cell in my body. All my days are written in his book (see Ps. 139:16). He alone has the power to heal me and keep me healthy if it is his will. He will work regardless of my positive thinking or faith—his healing work does not depend on me. My trust should be in God's good plan for my family and me—whatever that plan is—rather than in my ability to stay positive.

Battling cancer is very stressful. When I was told that my attitude was a factor in whether or not I survived, it felt like even more pressure. It made me feel that I was somehow responsible for the success or failure of the cancer treatment. If I had a bad day, if I was wrestling through fear and the reality of my mortality and shortened life expectancy, was I somehow making it more likely that my children would grow up without their mom? The message seemed to be that if my illness ended badly, it was my fault because I didn't believe that I would be healed. I don't believe this to be true or biblical.

Your friend may not be as sensitive about this as I was. But, just in case, don't put this pressure on your friend. Encourage her to be hopeful as long as the doctors are offering that hope. (If your friend has been told there is nothing more that can be done medically, that is a different discussion. We'll address this in chapter 12.) But please do not connect her positive attitude to a particular outcome. There are no guarantees in the world of cancer except this: God is good, and he is in charge. Encourage your friend to put her trust in him rather than in her ability to stay positive.

"None of us are promised tomorrow. I could get hit by a bus and die next week!"

It's true that we don't know how long we have on this earth. But unless you are also battling a life-threatening illness, you are not facing this truth in the same way your friend is right now. You probably don't look at your children and wonder if you'll see them grow up or if you'll hold their babies. You probably haven't thought about whether it would be better for your family if you die at home or at a hospice facility, and you probably haven't checked how many more years are left on your life insurance policy. So please understand that your friend is facing her mortality in a way that you are not.

This might be difficult for your friend to discuss. She may be afraid that it will upset you, or these emotions may be too raw for her to talk about. Be sensitive and listen carefully for clues to how she is feeling. If you are a close friend, you might ask gently how she is feeling about her future or if she is struggling with fear. Tread carefully and prayerfully in this area, and God may use you to bring comfort and encouragement to your friend. We'll talk more about this in chapter 9.

The husband of a cancer-fighter summarized how not to say the wrong thing this way: "Just don't be weird." But what if, despite your best efforts, things get weird? Chances are, you'll experience awkward moments when attempting to support your friend. You'll say the wrong thing. Maybe, after reading this chapter, you've realized that you've already gotten it wrong. Don't be afraid to keep trying. Your friend knows that it's hard. She knows that you don't know what to say. Reaching out and getting it wrong is still better than not reaching out at all. When those awkward moments happen, apologize and move forward. Your friend will appreciate your continued efforts to love her compassionately.

Questions for Reflection

1. Are you tempted to ask inappropriate questions or to share religious platitudes with your friend? What are some practical steps you can take to be a better listener?
2. When you do speak, what are some more helpful words of comfort you could share? (Resource 4.1 has some verses you may consider sharing when the time is appropriate.)

ACTION STEPS TO CONSIDER

☐ Say less. Listen more. Be willing to sit with your friend through silence, tears, or whatever she needs to say.

☐ Ask questions that are caring and appropriate and that seek to understand, rather than fix, your friend's problems.

☐ Avoid religious platitudes and clichés. Be patient with your friend's grief and with how the Lord is working in her life. Resource 3.1: A Biblical View of Suffering will help you to walk more thoughtfully with your friend through hardship.

☐ Keep your focus on your friend rather than relating her situation to your own experience or feelings.

☐ Don't give advice, minimize her pain, or share discouraging information. Speak words of encouragement, support, and comfort.

Diagnosis

A Stressful Beginning

I sat in the hallway of the Breast Center right outside Dr. Pope's office, alternating between checking my watch and checking my phone, and fidgeting in the small, uncomfortable chair. Where was he?!? I had only been waiting a few minutes, but I didn't know how much longer I could do this. I was surrounded by flyers and bookshelves full of books about surviving breast cancer. But I didn't have breast cancer. And there were certainly no books on those shelves about the rare cancer I'd been diagnosed with forty-eight hours earlier.

As I waited, I watched Dr. Pope walk in and out of his office a couple of times, glancing sideways to make sure I was still sitting alone. I tried to read his expression—was it good news or bad? Good news would be a bright spot in a very dark week. I might be able to eat and sleep again. If it was bad news, I would be unlikely to see my thirty-fifth birthday. The stakes were high.

I was tempted to stand up and walk into his office, but I knew I had to wait. My husband was finishing his work at a nearby surgery center and then joining me in Dr. Pope's office for the results of that day's PET scan and breast MRI. I was fresh out of the MRI machine down the hall, the bandage from the IV still on my arm. It had been only two days since the phone call with the cancer diagnosis. The first step in drafting a game plan was determining whether or not the cancer had spread elsewhere.

Finally, a text came from my husband. He was on his way. I tried to breathe and imagined how the meeting would unfold. Would we go in and sit down? Would the doctor look us in the eyes, pause, and then deliver the news? Would I fall apart if the news was bad? Would I fall apart if the news was good?

I listened to nurses in the next room talk on the phone, and I kept flashing back to the numerous phone conversations I'd had with medical personnel in the past two days. Were they on the phone with other newly diagnosed women? Setting up more PET scans and MRIs? I wondered how the women on the other end of those phone calls were holding up. Anything to take my mind off this excruciating wait.

By the time my husband walked in, still wearing scrubs, I was so scared I could barely stand up. Someone let Dr. Pope know he'd arrived, and the doctor poked his head out of his office and invited us in. My husband went first, and I trailed behind him, forcing my feet to take those heavy steps. There was no dramatic moment. No pause as he looked into our eyes. As we were still walking in, I heard him say to my husband, "The PET looks good." And, for the first time since my biopsy five days earlier, I could breathe.

The Three Phases of Cancer

Like many things in life, cancer has a beginning, a middle, and an end.

First comes the diagnosis and its immediate ramifications, both physical and emotional. Shock, sadness, and fear accompany this initial diagnosis. Further medical tests then determine the extent and severity of the cancer, and these test results lead to a treatment plan. A second opinion may be sought during this time. Medical appointments and responding to expressions of support occupy most of the new cancer patient's time at this stage.

The middle phase consists of receiving treatment to fight the cancer. This treatment may include surgery, chemotherapy, immunotherapy, and/or radiation. The phase lasts anywhere from weeks to years.

In cases in which cancer returns, these diagnosis and treatment phases may repeat multiple times.

Finally, treatment ends and the patient moves on as a survivor—or, in the case of incurable cancer, enters end-of-life care.

In this chapter, we will explore the first phase of your friend's cancer journey and how you can support her in the early days of the diagnostic process.

A Traumatic Emotional Experience

I don't have to explain how traumatic it is to hear that you have cancer. You've probably put yourself in your friend's shoes and imagined how she must feel. What surprises me is how long the pain associated with that moment lasts. Several years later, writing about that day still makes my heart race. Every survivor I've spoken with talks about Diagnosis Day in vivid detail: the setting, the doctor's words, the shock, the tears, the endless phone calls. It was a defining event in each of our lives.

Two days after my diagnosis, I underwent tests to determine whether or not the cancer had spread. For those two days, I barely ate or slept. Stress consumed me. I celebrated my thirty-fourth birthday the day after the diagnosis and wondered whether I'd live to see my thirty-fifth. At times I felt hopeful, buoyed by God's grace, confident in his faithfulness, and determined to fight in his strength. But I also had moments of fear, sadness, and dread of what lay ahead for my family and me.

My friends listened with compassion and courage as I struggled with my mortality. They gathered to pray for me as we all wept together. They didn't shy away from the difficult discussions I needed to have about the possibility of death. They didn't try to rush me through grief, even though I'm sure they were uncomfortable and upset. My friends suffered as they shared those excruciating moments with me. But I needed them there to join with me in those hard places of sadness and fear.

Dealing with Uncertainty

One of the most difficult aspects of the diagnostic phase is the uncertainty that reigns between hearing that you have cancer and developing a game plan to fight it. For some, this process takes just hours—for others, it may be weeks or even months of testing, research, and experts. During the time it takes to gain a clear diagnosis, prognosis, and treatment plan, the uncertainty is almost unbearable. It's hard to cope when you don't yet know exactly what you are facing.

When Crystal met with an oncologist after a breast cancer diagnosis, her prognosis was unknown. Many aspects of her case pointed to a favorable prognosis, but the biggest tumor was touching her chest wall. The oncologist told Crystal that he wasn't sure how it was going to go. The outcome depended on how well the tumors—and especially the biggest one—responded to chemotherapy. She had to wait through twelve weeks of chemo for tests and further assessment. The uncertainty of her diagnostic phase lasted for months.

In the days following my diagnosis, I needed my friends to understand the gravity of what we were facing and the horrors of this disease. I struggled to comprehend my new and unexpected situation. I grappled with the reality of being diagnosed with a life-threatening illness and what it meant for my young children, my husband, and me. Yes, I would soon prepare for the fight and put on hopefulness and determination, but first I needed my friends to look with me into an uncertain future.

A New Form of Busyness

Do you have a busy week coming up? What if, next Monday, I told you to burn your to-do list and spend the next several days talking on the phone with family, friends, and medical professionals, sitting in waiting rooms and doctors' offices, traveling to get second and third opinions, researching the cancer you've just been diagnosed with, responding to thoughtful notes, emails, texts, and messages, and trying to discern which of the many offers of help you've received are genuine? And don't forget to buy a wig, have surgery to get a port placed in your chest,[1] take family photos before you lose your hair, think through what your family will need for the next six months, and frantically get as much of it done as you can. This is what the week of a cancer diagnosis feels like.

The three weeks between my diagnosis and the start of chemotherapy swirled with activity. Once we determined that the cancer hadn't spread, I began sleeping and eating again. Phone calls with my medical team seemed unending, and when I wasn't on the phone I was responding to messages from concerned friends. The to-do list I originally had for the week was trumped by a cancer to-do list that seemed unending. We traveled twice for medical opinions to Little Rock, Arkansas, and Houston, Texas. I tried to finish my Christmas shopping and wrapping. I lined up help for my kids and me during my first week of chemo. But it was hard to focus on the logistics of what needed to be done when my brain was muddled by fear and grief.

How You Can Help

Two weeks after my diagnosis, I wrote this CaringBridge post as I waited to meet with my oncologist at MD Anderson the next day:

> November 9, 2010: As I anticipate meeting with an oncologist for the first time and starting chemo as early as next week, it is all becoming more and more real. I'm so thankful for everyone's prayers and encouragement—it really makes a difference. When I start feeling sad or anxious, it brings me comfort to know that someone, somewhere is probably praying for me at that moment. The Lord has been bringing letters, emails, guestbook messages, etc. along at just the right moments when I need them. He is truly my Sustainer, and he has a lot of helpers!

You can't fix your friend's sadness or anxiety. You can't make that first oncology appointment any easier. But you can be a vital link in her support chain during those difficult days. The Lord will use you just as he used my friends.

Your friend needs you to be present with her in this hard time. Remember—shock and grief characterize this beginning phase. Your friend may seem scattered and unfocused. She's probably struggling to concentrate. She may be sad and weepy, or limp throughout these weeks in a fog of shock. She may feel strong, hopeful, and determined. She may swing between the extremes of all these emotions from one minute to another. Wherever your friend is emotionally right now, meet her there with support. This can be difficult if you're also feeling shocked and saddened by her diagnosis. You may need to vent to a friend who is further toward her outer circles. Have a good cry and pour your heart out to the Lord. Then grab a box of Kleenex and go comfort your hurting friend.

Your friend may be overwhelmed by corresponding with her supporters and passing along updated information after her medical tests and appointments. Perhaps you could offer to communicate with others on her behalf. With her permission, set up a website or social media page in order to streamline communication. CaringBridge websites are a great tool for keeping loved ones updated. They enable friends and family to request email or text notifications of new posts, lessening the burden on your friend to remember who needs the latest information.

If your friend will lose her hair during chemotherapy, consider arranging (and even paying for) a family photo shoot for her during this busy time. In the midst of so many urgent details, this never would have risen to the top of my own to-do list, but a group of friends arranged this for me. I cherished taking those photos with my family before losing my hair.

One word of caution: instruct the photographer to ask which family groupings or arrangements the family wants. Your friend might want individual photos with each of her kids. Or she may not. When our family was photographed prior to my chemotherapy, the photographer asked if she could take photos of just me. All I could think was that she was taking the photos that would be on display at my funeral. I didn't ask for those, and I would rather have just had photos of me with my husband and each of my kids. I would have also liked photos of my husband with each of the kids. When she didn't suggest those, it felt like the photo session was all about preparing for my possible death. Even still, I was so thankful to have those family photos before losing my hair!

This is also a good time to get your friend and her helpers

ready for the fight ahead. If possible, appoint someone to field all the offers of help and to assign tasks to friends. This takes a huge weight off your friend's shoulders as she's feeling overwhelmed! Before she starts treatment, ask her to show you where her cleaning supplies are. Ask about her family's dietary restrictions and set up a meal calendar. Ask her for family recipes you can distribute to those who bring a meal. Offer to go shopping for wigs or hats if she will lose her hair. This might also be a good time to shop for comfy pajamas and, if she's facing a mastectomy, button-down tops.

Just as I sat holding my breath outside Dr. Pope's office, this diagnostic phase might feel like a never-ending held breath for your friend. She will eventually take the next breath. Be patient—don't rush her or try to talk her out of feeling scared or overwhelmed. Breathe for her. Comfort her. Encourage her with your compassionate support. Once a plan solidifies and treatment begins, rally the troops and surround your friend with hopeful, positive cheerleaders. Put on your fighting gloves and lace up your work boots—a long road lies ahead of your friend, and she needs her team with her.

Questions for Reflection

1. What emotions did you feel when you heard that your friend has cancer? How do you think she's feeling? How is she expressing these emotions? Is she openly emotional or more reserved?

2. Which of the specific ways of supporting a friend in the diagnostic phase stood out to you as something that God is asking you to do for your friend? Write them down on pages 243–44, along with a plan to put the ideas into action.

ACTION STEPS TO CONSIDER

☐ Listen with compassion and courage if your friend wrestles with her mortality and the uncertainty that the diagnosis brings. Remember not to assume that you know how she's feeling—ask questions and listen well.

☐ Provide a safe place for her grief and fears about cancer, treatment, and the possible long-term implications.

☐ Understand her shock, lack of focus, and difficulty concentrating. Lend a hand with logistical details to ease her burden.

☐ If she will lose her hair, make arrangements with a photographer to gift her with a family photo session. Offer to help her shop for wigs, scarves, and/or hats.

☐ Consider how you can ease the burden of communicating updates to her family and friends—perhaps by setting up a website or social media page (such as Caring Bridge.com).

☐ Rally support and make sure that she knows she has a team of cheerleaders ready as she begins treatment.

Your Friend as a Sick Person

Understanding Physical Needs

After my second round of chemotherapy, I sat in the treatment room of the oncology clinic, waiting for the results of my blood tests. I knew that my counts would be low, but I still expected to attend my four-year-old's preschool Christmas program the next day. I planned to compensate for my low white blood cells and increased risk of infection by arriving early and sitting alone in the balcony. I would capture video and happy memories of my son ringing his jingle bells on the steps of the sanctuary with his fellow preschoolers and then leave quickly. I had missed the book-character parade the previous month due to appointments in Houston, and I was *not* missing the Christmas program.

The nurse walked toward me, report in her hand and a grim look on her face. She showed me the numbers and explained two areas of concern: my white blood cells were virtually non-existent (which I expected), and my red blood cells were low enough to require a transfusion (which I did not). As she delivered the next piece of news, she didn't realize how devastating the blow was: I had to report to the infusion center the next morning for a blood transfusion.

I argued and begged and pleaded. Could we wait and see if my red blood cells rebounded on their own? Could the transfusion be delayed a day? Could it start at noon? The answer to all my questions was no. There was no way around it. I would miss the Christmas program and trade it for a beige recliner and a couple of bags of red blood cells at the infusion center. Huge sobs shook my body. I didn't care that I was making a scene in front of dozens of people in the treatment room. My life was feeling more and more out of my control, and I hated feeling powerless.

Losing Your Health

Cancer is physically devastating in many ways. If the tumor hasn't made your friend feel rotten, the treatment probably will! Whether it's nausea, hair loss, fatigue, or surgery—or all of them combined—the physical implications of cancer hit hard. In addition to these side effects, your friend is adjusting to the change of her health status and possibly changes to her life expectancy.

I remember feeling confused about my new and unexpected status as a sick person. In the past, filling out a medical history had been a breeze. I had no interesting medical history, no previous surgeries, and nothing but three uneventful pregnancies to report. And even when they told me I had cancer, I didn't feel sick. Could I really have a rare, life-threatening illness? It didn't seem possible.

Then the treatments made me sick. I hated being sick. It was humiliating to be weak and tired. It was frustrating to lie in bed while others cared for my children and my home. Before cancer, taking a nap was a rare and delectable luxury. But cancer ruined naps for me. For years afterward I never took naps, because curling up under the covers in the middle of the day no longer felt like a treat—it felt like a prison, bringing back painful memories of my time as a sick person.

The cancer diagnosis not only rattled my identity, it also uprooted my assumptions about my life expectancy. Before cancer, I never questioned whether I would see my kids graduate from high school, hold my grandbabies, or grow old with my husband. All of a sudden, I couldn't even listen to my friends talk about parenting teenagers. It felt foolish to look that far into the future.

Shortly after my diagnosis, I chatted with another mom from my son's school at a social gathering, and she asked what our plans were for educating our son long-term. I said the first thing that popped into my head: "I may homeschool him down the road, you know, if I'm still alive." As soon as I saw the horrified look on her face, I knew that I needed a better filter between my thoughts and my mouth! But at that time, I couldn't handle thinking or talking about the future. The uncertainty was too painful and too fresh. I was still adjusting to the implications of my new reality as a woman with cancer.

Losing Your Hair

When you know that the chemo dripping through your IV tube will cause your hair to fall out, you have two options: shave it and get it over with, or hold onto your hair as long as you can while watching it fall out by the fistful in the shower and waking up to giant clumps of it on your pillow. Both options are equally valid and understandable. And, while I didn't want to be bald any longer than necessary, I opted for the first choice. My children were young, and my entire situation felt so out of my control that I chose to grab control of the one thing I could. I wanted to choose the day I would lose my hair. I wanted to give my children some warning. One night during my first round of chemo, as I tucked them into their beds and crib, I told them, "Mommy is going to have a new haircut tomorrow! I'll get to wear my new wig and some fun hats!" I forced a smile as I tried to be upbeat and reassuring.

Once they were asleep, I sat down in my bathroom and leaned forward so my head was over the tile floor. My husband used scissors and then a razor to rid me of my hair. I would be bald for the next several months, and it would be years before I'd have shoulder-length hair again. I didn't cry. I was sad, but the tears wouldn't come. I stared in the mirror and marveled at how much I looked like my brother. Then I pulled on a knit cap and left the room—I didn't want to stare at my reflection any longer.

Your friend will choose whether or not to wear a wig. Most women don't enjoy wearing wigs—they're uncomfortable and scratchy and feel weird. In the summer, they're dreadfully hot. But your friend may feel that there's no good choice. Imagine walking around in a winter hat in the summer. Then imagine walking around bald in the summer, seeing the pitying glances of strangers and the confused stares of children. Not an easy choice to make, right?

Being bald can make you feel weak, vulnerable, humble, and different. It immediately sets you apart from others. As a bald cancer patient, you realize the difficult emotions that you trigger in others. And if you wear a wig, the polyester netting and Velcro straps dig into your temples and remind you that nothing in your world is normal—and that it won't be for a long time.

I wore a wig every time I left the house. I had two reasons for this: my kids were young, and I didn't want them to deal with questions from their peers. I know several other moms of young children who made the same decision. My friend Crystal's six-year-old daughter wanted Crystal to wear a wig every time her young friends came over. She was terrified of her friends seeing her mom's bald head!

Another important reason I wore a wig is that I'm vain. This isn't true of all women who wear wigs—but it's true of me! When I was out, I wanted to look and feel normal. I didn't want to cope with the stares or the questions or the pity. I just wanted to take my kids to the park or to buy groceries like a normal mom.

My wig was fabulous, and it fooled everyone who didn't know what I was going through. I've never gotten so many compliments on my hair—it was always shiny and perfectly in place! If your friend doesn't have the resources to get a high-quality wig and you know that she'd like to have that option, consider rallying a group of friends to pitch in for a wig fund. In my area of the country, you can buy a high-quality wig for around $500, and there are many wig shops that offer a discount for chemo patients. Do whatever you can to help her get a wig that makes her feel beautiful if she decides to wear one. It makes such a difference!

You should emotionally prepare for the first time you see your friend after she loses her hair. It will be startling to see your friend looking like a cancer patient. Even if she wears a wig, the difference will probably be striking and upsetting to you. It may trigger memories of a grandparent or another friend who died of cancer. It may stir fears that you have for your friend and her future.

If you carry emotional baggage related to your friend's baldness, let me encourage you to process that before you see her. Sit and let those emotions and memories flood over you. Cry it out. Pray through your feelings. Ask the Lord to strengthen you as you support her. If you have young children, prepare them as well. Talk with them about your friend's hair loss and how they should respond. When you see your friend, be prepared to smile and to be positive and strong with your support. Tell her she looks beautiful. She needs to hear it.

It will be years before your friend's hair is back to normal. It may grow back with a different color or texture than before and may never look the same as it did before cancer. She may grieve the loss of her hair for years—not just at the time that she loses it. And she may struggle with guilt over this ongoing sadness. Don't be surprised if she seems more upset about her hair than about some of the bigger events like getting a port. Listen and let her grieve. Don't try to compare how big or small her concerns seem to you.

At first, I was thrilled when my hair came back in. I didn't care that it was super-short, dark brown, and curly—so different from my long, straight, dyed-blond hair before cancer. I was alive, and I had hair! Best feeling ever! But, a few months later, I was still stuck with short hair. I missed my long hair. I missed fitting in with other women my age and matching their hairstyles. I missed having a choice about what my hair looked like. I watched with jealousy as other women carelessly flipped their hair over their shoulders or grabbed a hair tie from their wrists to put their hair up on a hot day. Then I would feel guilty about being jealous. I'd feel guilty about wishing for longer hair. I didn't talk about it much, because it felt superficial and ungrateful to complain about having short hair. But it was a loss I needed to grieve.

Losing Your Breasts

I sat in Sunday school and looked around the large circle of chairs filled with my brothers and sisters in Christ. I'm sure that the lesson was important and riveting, but that morning all I could think about was how the other women could dress to complement their figures. One wore a low-cut sundress. Another's blouse showed off her curves. I thought of how I looked in the mirror that morning, trying to find an outfit that would camouflage my lopsided chest.

To save my life, I underwent a single mastectomy at the

end of my chemotherapy and radiation treatments. Unable to have reconstruction at the time of surgery, I didn't think much of it. Maybe I wouldn't bother with it. After all, I was thankful to be alive and wanted to spend time with my family. I had no plans to voluntarily give up more hours and days to another surgeon's waiting room or an operating room. I accepted my identity as a self-nicknamed uniboober. I had a prosthesis made (a.k.a. my "foob") and learned to buy shirts that didn't reveal how my chest slanted outward on one side and went straight down on the other. Shopping goes quickly when you walk into a store and rule out two-thirds of the tops immediately. Just show me to the turtlenecks, please!

Yes, I tried to have a sense of humor about my situation. I have a few hilarious stories to tell—there's a middle-aged male TSA agent out there who's probably still blushing about my prosthesis! But I needed my friends to understand that, on the inside, I was grieving. The months after my mastectomy when I was still bald were especially difficult. I felt like a broken, scarred shell of the person I used to be, at least on the outside. I didn't feel sexy or feminine anymore, and I feared it would impact my marriage.

After two years of good health, I decided I was ready to face the operating room again and sought reconstructive surgery. It took seven months and three surgeries to put me back together again. I needed meals and help with my kids yet again, and it felt selfish—more selfish than when I had no choice during the cancer surgery and treatments. But I've never regretted saying goodbye to that constant physical reminder of cancer.

Your friend may not be in the same situation I was. It's unusual these days for a woman to undergo a single mastectomy, but there are times when reconstruction goes awry or the treatment plan forces her to delay reconstruction. If your friend has immediate reconstruction, her breasts still won't look the same as before. I hope my experiences shed light on how it feels to cope with these physical changes. Remember, the scars will be a daily reminder of what your friend has endured. She'll need to grieve the loss of her breasts and the changes to her body. This grief may be complicated by guilt.

You can help your friend after her mastectomy by practicing modesty, especially around her and her husband. Understand that she may feel insecure or unsure about her changed body, and you can respect her feelings by not flaunting what you have. Be sensitive to her feelings and be a judgment-free place for your friend to share her thoughts about her post-cancer body.

Can we talk about elective plastic surgery for a moment? (If you haven't had it and never will, you get to skip this paragraph.) I'm so happy for you if you've gotten the augmentation or reduction that you've always wanted, but please be cautious discussing your surgery with your friend. When I was diagnosed, a friend of mine had recently undergone a breast reduction. We hadn't seen each other yet, and she hadn't told me about her surgery. In our second or third conversation after my diagnosis, she gently let me know that I might notice something different about her when I saw her. She acknowledged that she felt weird about it, considering what I was going through. Her acknowledgment was all I needed from my friend to help me *not* feel weird about it. When other friends hid their plastic surgery from me, or when they gushed to me about every detail, I felt misunderstood and unloved. Please, don't ever compare your elective plastic surgery to your friend's reconstructive surgery. They are not the same. Not even close.

Losing Your Mind

You may feel skeptical if you hear your friend talk about chemobrain. She feels forgetful and foggy-headed—who doesn't, right? We're all stressed and getting older, and those neurons don't fire as quickly as they used to.

Let me assure you that chemobrain is real. I still struggle with memory issues, lack of focus, and the inability to multitask. It causes embarrassment and even feelings of frustration and failure. When I talk to other survivors who endured chemo, many of them are experiencing the same symptoms, even years later.

Chemobrain as a survivor is annoying, but it was much worse during my months of treatment. I experienced a thick mental fog each time I received chemo. The fog grew thicker and lasted longer with each round. I couldn't concentrate on anything—not books, movies, or even my beloved football games on TV. During my sixth round of chemo, a friend was driving me home from the hospital after I'd had my pump disconnected, and I started to say something. I startled her so badly that she actually jumped in her seat! I'd barely uttered a word over the course of several days, so she didn't expect me to start talking. I had no idea it had been that bad. Looking back, I appreciate how my friend embraced my need for quiet and rest.

When your friend's chemobrain is at its worst (typically during chemo and the days immediately following), you may need to be content with her silence, as my friend was with me. You can also support her by validating her concerns and not dismissing them. Help her find coping mechanisms to deal with her cognitive struggles—the reminder app on my phone is a lifeline for me. Forgive her when she forgets your birthday, and laugh in all the right places when she tells you that funny story . . . for the third time.

Other Physical Challenges

In addition to the loss of her identity as a healthy person, her hair, her breasts, and her mind, your friend will likely face many other physical challenges as a result of her cancer and treatment. These struggles are not only physical; they often become emotional struggles as well, as her physical issues cause her life to be unpredictable. She may feel helpless and even hopeless at times. You can support her by understanding the treatment she's receiving and how the side effects impact her daily life and future.

For me, the most difficult side effects of treatment were fatigue, nausea, and a suppressed immune system. During chemo and the week after, I was so tired. I've been Momma Tired. I've been First Trimester Tired. I've been College Senior Up All Night Writing a Research Paper Tired. Add all those together and double it, and that's what Chemo Tired feels like.

Thankfully, we have fabulous medications for fighting nausea now. That hasn't always been the case. A friend of mine received chemotherapy for breast cancer fifteen years ago. She would vomit as she entered the chemo room, even before receiving the chemo, because her body was responding with fear and dread of the nausea that was inevitable over the next several days. But the anti-nausea drugs also have side effects. I'll spare you the details, but let's just say that if you want to throw in a bottle of stool softeners with the next gift you give your friend, they won't go to waste.

For me, the nausea didn't cause vomiting—I just couldn't eat. It was hard to explain. Smells made it worse. Spicy foods, or even a nice savory dish, made it worse. During chemo I lived on breadsticks and apples. Some days I didn't eat at all.

One of the most dangerous side effects of most chemotherapy drugs is how they wipe out your bone marrow. Simply put, your bone marrow makes the red blood cells, white blood cells, and platelets your body needs in order to function properly. Most chemo patients will see drops in one or more of these blood cells following each round of chemo. The effects worsen as chemotherapy progresses, and the impact on the body accumulates over time. In my case, all three types of blood cells plummeted to dangerous levels, starting with my second round and worsening every round after that.

Low red blood cells cause fatigue, weakness, and nausea. (It's like chemo week on replay!) If they get extremely low, a blood transfusion is needed. Low platelets increase the risk of uncontrolled bleeding and are more difficult to treat, although transfusions are an option. Low white blood cells leave you susceptible to germs and unable to fight any infection or virus you may catch. Most patients receive injections to boost their white blood cells, but the injections can take a few days to work, and in the meantime the patient may need to avoid germ-ridden public places (such as preschool Christmas programs!). The injections often cause side effects, too, such as bone pain and flu-like symptoms.

This is the life of a cancer patient. Your health is unstable; life is unpredictable. Your body feels like it should belong to someone else. Infections land you in the hospital. Low blood counts require day-long transfusions. You experience side effects of the drugs that are treating the side effects of the chemo. Surgical complications require emergency surgery or bed rest. New tumor growth on a routine scan can cause a shift in the treatment and upend all the plans you had penciled on the calendar. (Pencil, always pencil. Cancer patients forget about using pens on calendars.) It's not easy being a sick person.

How You Can Help

Realize that there's more to the story.

Take time to understand how your friend is physically affected by cancer and the treatment she receives. People often assumed I was doing well most of the time because I looked well when they saw me. They didn't understand that when I wasn't feeling well, I didn't leave the house! Or sometimes I would spend the day resting so I would be able to leave the house for a short, planned outing. I tried desperately to act normally when I was out, because I didn't want to make people feel uncomfortable. I'd "paint" on eyelashes and eyebrows, wear a wig, get dressed, and put a smile on my face—but it wasn't my daily reality. The reality was a bald woman with no eyelashes, lying in bed or stumbling into a doctor's office for a blood transfusion. Try to avoid basing your assumptions on how your friend seems when she's out somewhere, as this is likely not a realistic or accurate perspective.

Invite her to sit down.

When you visit in person, make sure she sits down. Your friend may be too proud to ask you to come past the entryway in order to sit with her. But she's probably very tired and would appreciate having a seat while you chat.

Moms and kids, keep your germs at home!

I cannot stress this enough: if your children attend school or church with your friend's children, keep your sick kids at home. I understand the temptation to believe that your toddler with a low-grade fever is cutting teeth or that the green snot coming out of his nose is allergies. But your friend needs her kids to stay healthy. If she is receiving chemotherapy, she may not have the white blood cells to fight infection, and a small virus could land her in the hospital. Please be considerate and take extra precautions to protect her family. You may also consider communicating the importance of this to others whose children attend church or school with her kids. When a friend of mine received chemo, I posted regular reminders on our class Facebook page asking the parents to keep sick kids at home. And, of course, people should visit your friend only when they are healthy.

Research her illness and treatment, but be careful with your questions to her.

Take the time to understand the type of cancer your friend has and the implications of her diagnosis and treatment plan. What changes to her body will she endure? Hair loss, mastectomy, other cancer-removal surgery, reconstructive surgery, colostomy—all of these physical changes have long-term implications. Learn to speak the lingo and understand what your friend is facing, physically and medically.

Depending on how close you are to your friend, it may not be appropriate for you to ask for this information from her. You may need to head to the internet or other sources for your research, and you may need to provide the best support you can with incomplete information. Don't worry—the Lord will guide you!

Think carefully before commenting on the changes to her body or asking probing questions. Remember our discussion in chapter 4 about asking careful questions. If you weren't close enough friends to talk about her breasts before cancer, it's not appropriate to do so now. If she offers the information publicly, it might be okay to ask her how she feels about it. Ask an open-ended question and follow her lead. She may not want to talk about baldness or mastectomies today. Let her guide the conversation.

Acknowledge her grief.

Take the time to understand your friend's prognosis and the grief process associated with changes to her health and life expectancy. Your friend needs to grieve the loss of the expectations she had for her body and for her future. Do not rush her through this process. Recognize how her reality is permanently altered, and listen patiently to her feelings.

If there is a genetic component to her diagnosis, she may also struggle with fear for her children, grandchildren, and other family members. This is a common fear for breast cancer patients. Even without a genetic link in my case, it crosses my mind often that my medical history puts my loved ones at higher risk for a cancer diagnosis. The better your understanding of her grief, the better support you can provide her as she wrestles through these emotions.

Do not complain about your healthy body.

One way you can show consideration for your friend's grief process is to avoid complaining about your own body. News of your friend's mastectomy and reconstructive surgery should not be met with comments about your desire for breast implants (remember chapter 4?). If she loses weight while receiving chemo, don't tell her that you're jealous of her thinner frame. I know you would never intentionally hurt your friend with your comments, but sometimes when we don't know what to say, these comments sputter out of our nervous mouths. She would trade for your healthy, sagging breasts and love handles in a second. Limit your responses to remarks that communicate support and questions that seek a better understanding of her experience.

Do not give medical advice.

We talked about this in chapter 4, but it bears repeating. No matter how much research you do, please refrain from giving your friend medical advice. She has a team of doctors who have gone to school for many years to become experts in medicine and cancer. Let them be the doctors—you be the friend. Unfortunately, your friend will probably receive lots of medical advice. Others might even become pushy if their advice isn't heeded. Don't put your friend in the uncomfortable position of not taking your advice. If you have expertise in the field of oncology due to training or personal experience, it's fine to let her know that you'd be happy to share your experience with her, and then let her ask you for the information.

The physical losses that your friend will experience aren't the whole story, but they're an important piece of her grief puzzle. When you acknowledge the physical challenges she's facing, you give her freedom to grieve. This will also help you to see how her physical restrictions lead to the logistical needs we will discuss in the next chapter, and you'll be ready to provide the physical support your friend needs.

Questions for Reflection

1. What questions do you have about your friend's treatment or prognosis? Do you need to set aside your need for these answers, or is there someone you can ask? (Note: It is probably not appropriate to ask your friend or those closer to her for this information. The internet or a medically knowledgeable friend who is further removed from the situation might be able to help.)
2. If your friend will lose her hair, how do you think you will feel the first time you see her bald? Try to process some of these feelings ahead of time so that you can focus on supporting your friend when the moment comes.
3. What are the places where you see your friend or where your family members see hers? Remember to be aware of your family's health before they are around your friend or her family. Who else can you share this information

with on behalf of your friend? Make a note to repeat this reminder again at the start of cold/flu season.

4. What are the names of your friend's doctors and nurses? Write them down on page 245 and add them to your prayer list. Your friend will appreciate it if you know the names of doctors and nurses who she sees regularly, so that she doesn't have to explain who she's talking about every time.

ACTION STEPS TO CONSIDER

☐ Ask questions about how she's feeling and realize that you aren't getting the full picture when you see her out in public.

☐ Ask if she needs to sit down while you visit, so that you don't wear her out by standing too long.

☐ If you or your kids are sick, please stay at home! Communicate the importance of this to others on your friend's behalf.

☐ Learn about the side effects of her illness and treatment, both immediate and long-term. Learn to speak the lingo of her specific cancer and its treatment.

☐ Let her grieve the loss of her health and its potential impact on her life expectancy.

☐ Don't complain about your healthy body. Instead, listen as she talks about the changes to her body, ask questions, and offer support.

☐ Don't give medical advice. Let the doctors do the doctoring.

Everything That
Needs to Get Done

Tackling Logistical Needs

When Lisa's husband was diagnosed with leukemia, she needed to accompany him to Houston for treatment. They left their teenage son, Christopher, in the care of friends. Lisa's inner circle worked together to arrange transportation for Christopher to and from school and extracurricular activities. They took him to his own house on a regular basis, so he could relax and spend time with his cats. And, on one particularly traumatic day for the family, a friend made the decision to keep Christopher home from school and spent the day with him. The friend's attentiveness to Christopher's needs was an encouragement to Lisa. She could focus on her husband's needs in Houston, knowing that her friends were caring for Christopher back home.

Cancer is a new full-time job that your friend never expected or wanted. She will spend a lot of time in doctors' offices—or, more accurately, a lot of time in doctors' waiting rooms! She will need extra rest. She may require chemotherapy, which takes several hours at a time, or radiation, which requires short amounts of time daily for several weeks. She will need your help with tasks she cannot do because she either is physically unable or doesn't have the time.

While I received chemo, there were many weeks when I couldn't care for my children. I wasn't allowed to drive. I didn't have the strength to cook, clean, or do laundry. And, the week after receiving chemo, I wasn't able to run errands or care for my family because of fatigue and the risk of infection.

Finances and insurance costs are another logistical concern for many cancer-fighters. Cancer is expensive. Depending on your friend's pre-cancer financial situation, her employment needs, and her insurance coverage, know that she may be incurring insurmountable costs, medical bills, and debt. Filing bankruptcy is not uncommon among people with cancer.

Fortunately, I was not the breadwinner for our family, and my husband continued to work. Our insurance covered my treatment with low out-of-pocket costs. Yet we still incurred thousands of dollars of unexpected expenses when I started a clinical trial in Houston. Over those months, we paid for childcare, plane tickets to and from Houston, and rental cars while I was there.

We needed an army of relatives, friends, and acquaintances to pull us through those months. Thankfully, we had more offers of help than we knew what to do with! Friends from our church, my parents' church, and my kids' school brought us dinner three times a week for eight months. One of my best friends took over the entire carpool to my kids' elementary private school in another county. Another bestie cleaned our house. My friends drove my kids to church and extracurricular activities, took them along on fun outings, and helped with our part-time homeschooling efforts. We received financial gifts, including checks, gift cards, frequent flyer miles, and an anonymous friend who paid one of our babysitters whenever she helped me with the kids. We never would have gotten through our cancer battle without the sacrificial service of our friends and family.

How to Offer Help
(and Let Her Tell You No)

I know you are eager to be a friendship rock star, like my friends were. You want your friend to know that you would do anything for her. But try not to say, "Let me know how I can help." This was mentioned by every single cancer survivor I spoke with, so I'm going to say it again.

Please do not say, "Let me know how I can help."

Even though you are sincere, your friend might not know how to take you up on this offer. Her life has been turned upside down, she has a new job that she didn't want, and she lacks the mental energy to coordinate her friends' efforts to help her. And, unfortunately, she will hear this comment from many people who don't really mean it. But I know that you mean it, so let's talk about how to offer help in a way that will enable her to accept it.

The best way to do this is to make your offers of help as specific as possible, while still giving her options. Here are some examples:

- "I'd like to bring you dinner next week. Would Monday or Thursday work?"
- "I'm going to the store tomorrow. Can I pick up bread, milk, or any other items for you?"
- "Can I keep your kids one day this week? I'm free on Wednesday or Friday."
- "I drive past your son's preschool on my way to work. Would it be helpful for me to drop him off for you on the mornings you're at chemo?"
- "I'd love to take care of any ironing you have—what time should I drop by to get it?"
- "I have some free time while the kids are at school this

week. If I came by for a few hours to do some cleaning, could you give me a list of your top priorities?"

- "Can I bring you lunch when you're at chemo? What sounds good to you?"
- "I know you've been receiving meals from friends, so I'd like to help you return any dishes the meals came in. May I stop by tonight at 7 to pick them up?"

The most helpful offers that my friends made were specific offers like these. When someone let me know a way she wanted to help or a particular day or time she was available, I could easily connect her offer with a need I had. And because my logistical needs were substantial and ongoing for several months, I especially needed people who could make a regular commitment. For example, someone offering to drive my child to preschool every Tuesday was much more helpful than someone offering to drive my child to preschool on just one Tuesday. I had a lot of Tuesdays to cover! So when friends made a weekly commitment, it was a huge blessing.

Once you've made your offer, give your friend the freedom to say no. She may be overwhelmed by the influx of meals. She may not be comfortable with having someone else clean her house or care for her kids. She may not be ready to accept help. She also may be clinging to any shreds of normalcy she can find. Respect her "no," but keep asking gently and specifically from time to time.

Food, Food, and More Food

When you take dinner to your friend with cancer, you have an opportunity to love her well and show your concern. Whether you make a homemade casserole or bring takeout, she's sure to appreciate it!

If you've been an adult for a while, you've probably already taken a meal to a new mom. But the needs of women with cancer are different. You're not dropping in on a smiling (but exhausted) woman cradling a newborn—in fact, you may not see your friend with cancer at all when you deliver a meal. Your friend's family may be receiving meals for several months, not just a few weeks. She may have strict dietary restrictions or preferences that need to be considered. Your friend's specific needs may vary, depending on her family situation and phase of treatment. If she is single or married with no kids at home, she doesn't need a large pan of lasagna. Consider splitting a dish into smaller portions so she can freeze some for later. If she's receiving chemo, ask if there are certain foods she needs to avoid or specific smells that trigger nausea.

A few things to remember when taking your friend a meal:

- Bring food in disposable containers so that your friend doesn't have to remember (or find the time) to return a dish. If you must take a dish that you need back, label it with your name and tell her that you'll stop by in a few days to retrieve it.
- Write out any meal instructions and attach them to the meal. Verbal instructions are easily forgotten! Label dishes with the date so that she can keep track of when leftovers need to be discarded.
- Consider bringing a package of paper plates and napkins so that she doesn't have to clean any dishes.
- Dinnertime can be hectic, so this is not the best time to sit and visit with your friend. Plan to drop off the meal and head out quickly so that she and her family can eat while the food is hot and continue with their evening routine.
- Ask if others have left dishes that need to be returned,

and offer to return them for her. She will appreciate your help with this task!

- Don't be disappointed if your meal is received by a family member and you don't see your friend. She may be resting, not feeling well, or having an emotionally difficult day. This is hard when you want to spend time with her, but remember that you are there only to serve her family.
- If you have young children, leave them at home or in the car if possible. This will help to protect her compromised immune system from possible germs. While I'm sure your children *never* pick their noses or lick the slide at Chick-fil-A, your friend will benefit from being exposed to as few people as possible. You should also let your friend know if anyone in your home is sick before going to her home.

If you want to go the extra mile, ask for her family's favorite recipes. I still remember when my friend Sarah made one of our family recipes. My children were thrilled to have something familiar! It happened to be one of my mom's recipes that I loved as a child, so it comforted me as well. No amount of nausea could keep me from the dinner table that night.

My friend Lesley shared a great story with me that is an exception to the "disposable dishes only" rule. A friend brought dinner to Lesley's family in a slow cooker and told Lesley that it was an extra one she uses specifically for taking meals. She let her know that she would be back to retrieve it soon, but it helped Lesley to know that her friend wasn't needing it right away to cook for her own family. It inspired me to want a ministry slow cooker, too!

You can also rally the troops for a freezer meal drive or a gift card drive. If you are connected through school, church, or a specific organization, ask others to make freezer meals or buy restaurant gift cards for her family. If her freezer space is limited, keep the meals in someone else's freezer and deliver them to her in small batches. These strategies work especially well during times when your friend doesn't want people coming to her house or when mealtimes become unpredictable.

And don't forget breakfast and lunch! While providing dinner is a huge help, your friend and her family are still eating two (or more!) other times a day. She will appreciate any healthy, ready-to-serve breakfast and lunch food you can provide. Not only will you save her time and energy, you will also save her money at the grocery store. When you're spending money on co-pays and deductibles, lower food expenses are a blessing! One of my friends regularly brought frozen, homemade blueberry pancakes that we could heat in the microwave and eat for breakfast. We also appreciated those who brought lunchbox supplies and snacks to stock our pantry.

Grocery shopping is another way you can serve your friend. Be sure to text or call when you are heading to the store to see whether there's anything she needs. When I was in treatment, two of my close friends kept envelopes of my money in their purses. They picked up groceries that we needed, figured out my total, and paid themselves out of my envelope. (I hope that they rounded up, because I bet that was a real pain!) When they ran out of my cash, I'd hand them more. This met a pressing need, since I was usually in Houston or didn't have enough white blood cells to be out in public. And if my husband went to the store, he came home with Ramen noodles, Pringles, and Mountain Dew!

Other Ways You Can Help

Logistical needs can be overwhelming, especially if your friend has young children or requires lengthy treatment. This list is a starting point to help you brainstorm ways you can help your friend or rally others to meet her unique needs:

- Give (or coordinate) rides to doctor appointments.
- Sit with her during treatment (if you're in her inner circle). Offer to write thank-you notes for her while you sit with her.
- Run errands for her, or drive her to run errands if she feels like getting out.
- Provide childcare.
- Drive her kids to school or to extracurricular activities.
- Take her kids along on fun outings.
- Offer to come over and help her kids with homework. This could be especially helpful if you know that there's a big project coming up. (School projects are hard enough under normal circumstances!)
- Clean her house. This may feel too personal to her—no one wants their friends seeing their filthy bathrooms! If she seems nervous about having friends clean, ask a few friends to share the cost of professional cleaning services.
- Mow her lawn and do yard work.
- Ask if her car needs an oil change, and take it to be serviced.
- Pick up her dirty laundry and return it clean and folded. If she feels weird about handing you her dirty underwear, offer to pick up loads of sheets and towels. You could stop by in the morning, strip the beds, take the sheets home to wash, and return later in the day to remake the beds.
- Iron clothes.
- Help with holiday shopping, decorating, and/or gift wrapping. Be sure to ask if there are certain aspects

of holiday preparation she'd like to do with her family. Maybe she'd love your help with decorating, but she and her family want to decorate the tree. Or you can wrap the gifts, but let her write the tags so that her family doesn't see a stranger's handwriting on Christmas morning.

- Respect her methods of parenting by maintaining similar boundaries and rules for her kids when you're caring for them. Ask her what things are most important to her when it comes to her children's routines, discipline, structure, and so on.

Help with medical appointments.

If you visit your friend during medical treatments, remember that you are there to bless and support her. If you are uncomfortable in a medical setting, this might not be the best way to serve your friend. You don't want her having to manage your emotions or discomfort! Be aware of whether she feels up to chatting or is becoming sleepy and needs rest. Bring a book with you if you are responsible for staying the entire time and driving her home. If you are popping in for a short visit, make sure she knows that you will leave if she needs a nap. Keep the visit brief so that she doesn't feel she has to entertain you.

Anticipate her unique needs.

In addition to the needs we have already discussed, try to anticipate needs that your friend may not be thinking of or may not have the courage to mention. Remember that anything you're doing for your household probably needs to be done for hers, and she may not be able to do it herself. When you clean out your flower beds and plant annuals in the spring, ask if her flower beds could use some TLC as well. When it's time to sign up for snacks for an office holiday party, sign up for her and let her know that you'll grab them at the store and take them to the party. If you're checking to see whether your kids have snow boots and gloves that fit, remember that her kids may need those items, too.

Consider the financial impact.

Financial stress may be an issue for your friend, depending on her insurance coverage and work situation. If she or her husband need to take lengthy time away from work, if she is a stay-at-home mom who suddenly needs a nanny, or if she has a high deductible for her health insurance, she could suddenly find herself in a difficult situation. Take some time to carefully ask about her financial situation and how you can help. Asking for money can be humbling, so these questions should be asked by a close friend and with great sensitivity. If help is needed, consider setting up a fundraising website or organizing a local fundraiser. Also, encourage your friend to ask for help from a social worker or patient advocate at her doctor's office. They can point her to resources and organizations that provide support for families walking through cancer.

Coordinate logistics for her.

If you are a close friend or a highly organized person, offer to coordinate the help of her larger circle of friends and acquaintances. Your friend does not have the energy to sort through offers of meals, assign dates to people, and make sure that she doesn't get three lasagnas in a row. You can offer to coordinate meals for her, using one of the many free sign-up tools online (my favorite is mealtrain.com). Make sure to ask about any dietary restrictions or preferences and communicate these to the volunteers. If your friend prefers to not have people in her home when she's feeling ill, you can arrange for the meals to be dropped off with a neighbor or in a cooler on her porch.

Start by asking your friend to send out a mass email or a post on social media stating that all offers of help should be sent to you. In addition to meals, you may also help to coordinate housecleaning, transportation, childcare, and other logistical needs during her treatment.

When Lisa's friends jumped in to care for her son, their attentiveness to her family's needs demonstrated their love and concern. They were probably inconvenienced at times as they shared Lisa's burden and freed her to focus on her husband's needs in Houston. No one friend could meet all the logistical needs created by Lisa's husband's diagnosis and treatment. In this chapter, we've covered a lengthy list of tasks that your friend may need help with. We're about to discuss many other emotional and spiritual ways to care for her. Remember that you will not be doing all these things, even if she needs them all. You are one link in her support chain. But, as you take part of your friend's load and place it on your own back, you will give her a little extra time and space to focus on her healing or caregiving. She will feel loved by you and cared for by the Lord as you meet her tangible needs.

Questions for Reflection

1. Think through your friend's week. What are her weekly responsibilities? Which of these might she be unable to do right now?
2. Think through your weekly schedule. Where do your responsibilities overlap with your friend's in a way that makes it simple for you to help her? Are there regular weekly commitments you can make? You can use the calendar on page 246–47 to coordinate.
3. Who else can you rally to help with your friend's

logistical needs? What is the best way for you and your group of friends to organize yourselves to meet her needs?

4. Which seasons or holidays will fall during your friend's treatment? How can you help her at these special times—helping with holiday preparations, cleaning out closets at the end of the season, taking her kids shopping for winter coats or school supplies, and so on? A planning sheet is available on pages 248–49.

5. What unique circumstances does your friend face with regard to her logistical needs? How can you and her other friends address these needs?

6. What are some meals that you make often that are easily doubled? Plan to make more each time you prepare this meal so that you'll have some to share with your friend's family.

7. What are some favorite foods of your friend and her family? Use the meal planning sheet on page 250 to keep track of meal ideas and your friend's preferences.

ACTION STEPS TO CONSIDER

☐ Instead of saying, "Let me know how I can help," make offers that meet a specific need and then give your friend options for how or when to accept the help.

☐ Look for opportunities to make a weekly commitment, such as driving her child to school every Tuesday.

☐ Let your friend decline offers of help if she's not ready, but continue to gently and specifically offer your assistance.

☐ Take her dinner in disposable containers, along with breakfast, lunch, and snack items.

☐ Consider organizing a freezer meal or restaurant gift card drive or assisting with her grocery shopping.

☐ Find out if she has other needs, such as transportation, cleaning, laundry, childcare, yard work, or finances.

☐ Anticipate your friend's needs. Remember that everything you are doing for your household probably needs to be done for hers as well.

☐ If you provide childcare, respect your friend's parenting methods and keep the expectations and boundaries for her children as consistent as possible.

☐ Offer to coordinate the logistical support of others by spreading the word about what your friend needs and providing a way for others to volunteer.

Heart

Nurturing Emotional Needs

We sat on the pink rug in my daughter's room, our backs propped against the white dresser that doubled as a changing table. It was a few days after my diagnosis, and there were still many unknowns. As we watched my toddler play with her toys, my friend Lynette made promises that I hope she'll never have to keep. She and her husband committed to come alongside my husband if I didn't survive and to help him raise our children. Their family was ready to sacrifice in order to help our family get through the worst if it came. Her promises were specific, sincere, and heart-wrenching.

I can't imagine how difficult it was for Lynette to say those words out loud. But these were the words I most needed to hear as I struggled with the reality of my prognosis and my fears for my children's well-being. My friend was willing to tackle this difficult conversation and to soothe the fears in my soul.

Caring for your friend's emotional needs will be much more challenging than picking up her dry cleaning or dropping off a casserole. Her needs may vary from day to day—possibly even from hour to hour! I've given you an example of helpful words that Lynette spoke to me, but I need to qualify this story by saying that these words were helpful only because they were spoken by a close friend who heard me voice my fear that I may not survive. If I hadn't been wrestling with my mortality, her words would have felt intrusive and unsettling. There are no easy formulas here. But in this chapter, we'll tackle some of the difficult emotions your friend is feeling and will prepare you to offer compassionate support with listening skills, patience, courage, prayer, and lots of love.

What Is My Friend Feeling?

Your friend is not only battling cancer; she is battling difficult emotions such as grief, fear, isolation, anxiety, shock, and overwhelming stress. For me, wrestling through these emotions was more difficult than the physical struggles I endured. I had a team of doctors working on my physical issues, but it felt like the emotional work was up to me. And I didn't know where to start.

Cancer causes anxiety.

Your friend's fears will be specific to her situation, but here are examples of the fears I experienced:

- Fear of treatment side effects (e.g., hair loss, risk of infection, damage to internal organs, surgical procedures, fatigue)
- Fear of recurrence of cancer following treatment
- Fear of how the stresses of cancer and changes to my body would affect my marriage
- Fear of how my children would respond to the stress on our family
- Fear of financial problems
- Fear of receiving bad news at doctors' appointments
- Fear of making the wrong medical decisions

- Fear that I would be abandoned by friends who couldn't handle what I was going through
- Fear of making people uncomfortable or upset
- Fear of life never returning to "normal"
- Fear of death (and what that meant for my loved ones)

Cancer can be isolating.

Throughout my cancer treatment, I received an outpouring of support through countless cards, emails, and guestbook messages on my blog. I knew that many people were following my story and praying for me. And yet it felt like no one knew what it was like to be me. Traveling to receive treatment, spending hundreds of hours in medical clinics, and needing to avoid public places contributed to these feelings of isolation. I missed seeing my friends and family.

For the first several months of my battle, I didn't know a single survivor of angiosarcoma. I didn't know whether survivors even existed, so I wondered whether anyone had battled this disease and lived. It felt like I was the only one on the planet experiencing this particular trial. There was no one to say, "I know how you feel." I hope that your friend has someone in her life who has walked a similar road. But if your friend is battling a rare cancer or has unusual circumstances surrounding her treatment plan, her sense of loneliness due to isolation may be especially pronounced.

Cancer is overwhelming.

Having cancer felt like a full-time job—and I was busy enough before cancer! My time was consumed with doctors' appointments, treatment, rest, and communication with others (including responding to emails, notes, and phone calls from well-wishers, doctors, nurses, and those who were helping with logistical needs). When I was first diagnosed with cancer, the outpouring of support was wonderful. But I spent so much time replying to messages that I started to feel like I needed a personal correspondence secretary. Some people expressed their own horror and fear when they heard my diagnosis. I had very little time to process my emotions or to talk about them with others. I definitely didn't have time for other people's emotions!

Cancer feels like it's taken over.

Yes, your friend's life is mostly consumed by cancer right now. But cancer isn't her life. It doesn't define her. Her experience will shape her identity, but it isn't the whole of who she is. When you think of her and speak to her, remember that there is more to her than her cancer diagnosis. From time to time, ask about her family, her hobbies, her passions—whatever makes her unique. When you do, you acknowledge that there's more to her life than her current struggles. You might say, "I bet you feel like all you talk about is cancer these days. Is there anything besides cancer you'd rather talk about for a bit?"

This might feel strange, as if you're ignoring the elephant in the room when you talk about everyday life in the midst of your friend's battle. I remember a coffee date with my friend Lesley a couple of years ago. She was receiving high doses of chemo to battle metastatic cancer, but she was having a good day. We met at a coffee shop before picking up our kids from school and covered the typical mom topics: busyness, homework, extracurricular activities, and so on. It's not that we never talked about cancer—we talked about it almost daily. But that afternoon, she needed to be a normal mom having coffee with a friend.

Cancer brings the loss of more than just her health.

We've talked about some of these losses already: her expectations for the future, her short-term and long-term plans, her sense of predictability and control, and possibly her hair, breasts, and mind. In addition, many cancer-fighters feel like they've lost who they were before the diagnosis. My friend Samantha finds it difficult to see photos of herself from before her breast cancer diagnosis. She told me, "I don't even know that person anymore. She doesn't exist." When everything is different because of cancer—physically, emotionally, relationally, and spiritually—the feelings of loss are overwhelming.

Your friend is facing both actual losses and anticipated losses. Even if her prognosis is good, she may anticipate the possibility of recurrence and death. She may anticipate not being able to resume her normal activities after treatment or wonder if her marriage will be the same after a mastectomy. These anticipated losses must be grieved, just like the actual losses she's experiencing.

Reminders of the losses are everywhere. When I was sick, my daughter loved the book about monkeys jumping on the bed. I would read the story to her and fight back tears. As each monkey falls and hits his head, *Mama* calls the doctor. In another favorite book, Mama reads the bedtime story to the llamas in pajamas. Mama also rocks her baby and sings, "I'll love you forever." Mamas are everywhere in children's books. I wondered, *If I die, will someone take these books off her shelf? How many books will be left?*

Cancer brings grief.

Dealing with a cancer diagnosis is shocking, devastating, and life-changing. It forces you into the unnatural process of letting go of expectations you had for your life and your loved ones. And it requires you to consider your mortality. Grief is a process that takes time, and it will continue long after the medical treatment is finished. Your friend may not recognize it or acknowledge it yet, but she needs to allow herself the time and space to grieve her diagnosis and its possible implications for her life. She also needs your ongoing compassion, understanding, and listening ear as she moves through the grief process. We discussed physical losses that she's grieving in chapter 6, but remember that there are also emotional losses she's grieving, such as those we have talked about in this chapter.

You probably didn't need to be convinced that having cancer is hard. But I hope now you understand more of what's going on in your friend's heart. Let's dive into how you can walk with her through this difficult time.

A Framework for Supporting Your Friend

As you consider how to encourage a friend who is going through cancer or any other crisis, picture her in a large, dark, inescapable pit. How can you love your friend when she's in the pit?

You could shout down something encouraging, like "God has a good plan for your life!" and go along your merry way. (And your friend would wish she could get out of the pit and punch you in the face.)

You could throw yourself into the pit and curse God for putting both of you there. You could commiserate about how terrible the pit is and wonder what in the world God was thinking when he allowed your friend to fall into this pit. (Your friend wouldn't be alone, but she also wouldn't feel encouraged.)

Or you could jump down into the pit with her and hold her hand and pray with her. While acknowledging how difficult and sad and scary the pit is, you could gently remind her that the truth about God is just as true at the bottom of the pit as it is at the top. As you weep with her in the pit, together you could call to mind God's past faithfulness and his promise to redeem your life from the pit and to crown you with steadfast love and mercy (see Psalm 103:4). I call this last method the "This sucks, but God is good, and I love you" approach.

This sucks . . .

My parents taught me not to use that word. Sorry, Mom, but "Cancer stinks" just doesn't cut it. Your friend needs you to acknowledge the reality of her situation: her life has been turned upside-down and forever changed by the diagnosis of a life-threatening disease. If you fail to recognize this reality, you will lose credibility as a safe friend who understands what she's going through.

But God is good . . .

Proverbs 12:25 says, "Anxiety in a man's heart weighs him down, but a good word makes him glad." After you've cried together at the bottom of the pit for a while, gently remind your friend that God's promises are still true. God's Word is the anchor your friend must cling to while the storm rages around her. Speak the truth to her. Pray the truth with her. Write the truth on note cards for her, tape Scripture to her bathroom mirror, text Scriptures to her—whatever you can do to constantly keep God's promises in and on her mind. She is battling cancer, but she is also battling fear and despair—and is grieving. Those difficult emotions will be pushing the truth out of her mind, and you can help to push it back in. Remind her of God's goodness, faithfulness, power, love, provision, and peace!

You will probably struggle with when to stick with "this sucks" and when to move to "but God is good." Your friend may question God, question her faith, or struggle with anger and not want to hear about God's goodness. In those moments, you may wonder which is the more loving approach: to simply commiserate with her or to gently speak truth about the Lord into her heart. We've talked about being careful with our religious platitudes, and this is territory to tread carefully. The only advice I can give you is to pray. Before each text, before each phone call, before each visit, seek the Lord's wisdom. Ask him to guide your words and actions. He knows what your friend needs, and he will use you as an instrument of his love to her.

And I love you.

When I was diagnosed with cancer, one thing I found strange was that everyone started telling me they loved me. Not just family and close friends—people I never would expect to say those words were suddenly saying, "I love you." At first, it felt a little weird. Was I supposed to say, "I love you, too"? Or just say thanks? Were they saying it because they thought I was about to die? Were they pitying me? Did they really mean it?

But once I got used to it, I was comforted and encouraged to hear how many people loved me. They must have meant it, because I felt loved. And when you are facing difficult circumstances, it helps to feel loved!

You may or may not feel comfortable saying the words "I love you" to your friend. But you can communicate your love by letting her know that you're thinking of her often and praying for her. You can reassure her that you are in this fight with her. You can demonstrate your love by visiting her and serving her. All these expressions of love will communicate to your friend that you care about her and what she's going through.

I've developed this framework as I've struggled to find words for my friends who are suffering. Before cancer, I was heavy on the "God is good" approach to my friends' pain. You're hurting? Here's a verse! God is good—don't you feel better?! Now I understand that, while my friends need to hear this truth, they also need more. Practically speaking, my use of these three key phrases isn't always a text that says, "Wow, this sucks. Remember, God is good! And I love you!" Sometimes I spend time camped out on one thought before moving to the next. For example, if a friend receives bad news after scans, I might respond with, "I hate that you got such bad news today. I'm so sorry." She may need time to process before hearing the "God is good" part. The next day, I might text her again to say, "I'm so sorry you're going through this. Here are some song lyrics that have encouraged me when I'm hurting. I love you, and I'm in this with you."

With this basic framework in mind, let's talk about how you can care for your friend's difficult emotions. We'll discuss five ways you can love your friend as well as specific actions that will demonstrate your concern.

Love By Listening

The first and most important way to care for your friend emotionally is to listen well. Remember that everyone processes a cancer diagnosis differently. Don't compare your friend's reaction to her cancer diagnosis to someone else's. No matter how many people you have known with cancer—and even if you've survived cancer yourself—don't assume that your friend is feeling the same way. In fact, don't make any assumptions at all about how your friend is feeling. Ask questions and listen.

Your friend knows that you don't know what to say. And it's okay to say just that. She wouldn't know what to say if the roles were reversed. She's been diagnosed with a serious illness, and depending on her treatment and her prognosis, she may be dealing with major changes to her body, her lifestyle, and her life expectancy. You cannot fix this. Even if you could figure out the most perfect, profound, thoughtful words to say, your friend would still have cancer. You don't need to have answers or perfect words. Just sit with her and be a safe place where she can share her feelings when she's ready.

Love by Letting the Friendship Be One-sided

Remember, your friend is overwhelmed by the emotions we talked about. And, at the risk of sounding harsh (because I know it's tough when your friend has cancer), you need to remember that this isn't about you. Your friend may say or do things that hurt your feelings. Be prepared to extend grace and forgiveness.

Before my cancer diagnosis, I drove my half of a preschool carpool and an elementary school carpool. I offered to keep my friends' kids when they had hair appointments. I showed up with a latte when a friend's baby kept her up all night. But when cancer hit, my friendships all became one-sided. I didn't drive carpool. I didn't show up with lattes. And I certainly didn't keep anyone else's kids. I couldn't even care for my own!

This transition was hard for me and hard for my friends. I hated my new role as the needy friend. I knew that my illness was a burden for my friends. It was a burden they gladly carried, but it was tough on them, too. Instead of a having a friend they could call on, they had a friend who needed their weekly help. Our friendships weren't only one-sided from a logistical perspective, either; they were one-sided from an emotional perspective. I was simply trying to survive, drowning in the ocean of my raw emotions. I was barely able to talk with my husband and children about their feelings, so I was completely incapable of caring for the hearts of my friends.

Keep this in mind, and don't ask for or expect emotional support from your friend with cancer. She doesn't have it to give right now. You will be on the giving side of this one-sided friendship for a while. And that's yet another way that you can love her well. You will, however, need to process through your grief—especially if you're one of her close friends. Seek out a different friend, pastor, or counselor who has the emotional capacity to help you to process your feelings.

Love by Letting Her Grieve

Resist the temptation to rush your friend through her sadness, fear, and shock. I know that you hate to see her hurting. You want her to feel better physically and emotionally. But she needs to work through her feelings on her timetable. Let her know that you are hurting for her and with her.

Remember all those losses we've talked about? Her grief process may be lengthy and difficult. Acknowledge that you don't understand what she is going through. Resist the temptation to make comparisons between your friend's cancer and other hardships you have endured. Give her time to be sad. Be a safe friend who sits with her while she cries. Let her be angry if she needs to be.

While you let her grieve and make sure she feels heard, you will need to walk the fine line between encouraging her and disregarding her feelings. Whether she says it out loud or not, your friend is frightened. If she needs to talk about death, don't gloss over her fears by saying, "Oh, don't talk that way— you will be fine." Listen to her and let her talk about how she's feeling, even if you're uncomfortable. But, unless her doctors have told her the disease is terminal, she needs you to remain positive. Consider saying something reassuring, yet hopeful: "I know you're scared. If the worst happens, of course I will help your husband with the kids. But we're not to that point yet. You are beating this!"

Love by Leaving Room for Her Questions

Your friend may not package her feelings for you with pretty paper and a bow. She may be angry with God. She may question why this is happening and whether she can endure it. She may wrestle with the grief, isolation, fear, and lack of control that cancer brings to her life. You might not have answers to these struggles. That's okay.

First Thessalonians 5:14 says, "And we urge you, brothers, admonish the idle, encourage the fainthearted, help the weak, be patient with them all." When your friend is fainthearted, she needs your patience. Be willing to listen without giving advice or answers. Be comfortable with her questions. Leave room for uncertainty.

This isn't easy to do! We desperately want to solve the problems of those we love. You might think, "If she would just trust God more, or see things this way, she'd feel better." But you can't rush the work that God is doing in her life. You can trust him to use this trial for good in her life, even if you don't see it yet. In the meantime, be her safe friend who listens to her struggles without trying to have all the answers. We'll talk more about tough questions in chapter 9.

Love for the Long Haul

Make sure your friend knows that you are in this with her for the long haul. My cancer treatment lasted almost nine months. Then I dealt with the repercussions of the experience, both physical and emotional, for years following. When I was diagnosed with cancer, I experienced a huge outpouring of love and support. As time went on, I wondered if people would move on to the next crisis. I still needed them, but was I wearing them out? My friends let me know that they viewed our situation as a marathon, not a sprint. I felt secure and knew I had their support for as long as it took. Make sure that your friend knows you aren't going anywhere.

Cancer will change your friend forever. She will be different, even after her cancer treatment ends. Some of her friendships will survive this change, and others won't. If you want your friendship to last, you must be willing to walk through these changes with her. We'll talk more about this in chapter 13.

Tangible Ways to Care for Her Emotions

Your friend not only needs your understanding, she needs tangible reminders of your emotional support. Here are several ways to remind your friend of your love for her.

Contact her often.

Use text or email to communicate frequently that you are thinking of her and praying for her. Don't be afraid to call your friend—she will ignore you if she needs to. But text and email are a quick and nonintrusive way to remind her that you care. And, because life gets busy, consider setting a phone alarm or calendar entry to remind you to contact her on a daily, weekly, or monthly basis (depending on how close you are).

Let her off the hook.

When you write her a message, start off by saying, "You don't have to write me back." In the first few days after a cancer diagnosis, your friend is probably inundated with phone messages, emails, and texts. If she feels that she needs to respond to all of them, she will quickly become overwhelmed. During treatment, she may not have the energy to respond. She will appreciate you letting her off the hook whenever possible. This can apply to phone messages as well. Similarly, do not be offended when she doesn't respond, and don't let yourself wonder whether she wants to hear from you. Rest assured, she does!

Send her snail mail.

Write her encouraging notes—the kind you put a stamp on. Getting cards in the mail is a wonderful surprise in these days of electronic communication. When Becky's husband battled cancer, the stack of cards that they received served as a visual reminder of how many people were praying for them, and it eased her loneliness. Snail mail offers the added benefit of not requiring a response from your friend.

Stay informed.

Take the time to stay informed about what's happening medically with your friend. If she has a blog or posts updates on social media, that should be your first stop for information. And while "likes" are nice to see, she won't know if everyone who liked a post actually read it. Take the time to comment so she knows that you read her update and cared enough to respond.

A few years ago, I had lunch with a friend whose husband was fighting terminal cancer. We ran into someone she knew, and the other woman said, "How are you guys? Everything's still going great, right?" Actually, my friend had recently written a blog post sharing bad news, which this woman obviously had not read. It was awkward for all of us. If you haven't been staying informed, it's better to say, "I'm not up to date on how you are. How have things been going lately?"

Phrase your questions carefully.

Asking "How are you today?" feels less intimidating than "How are you?" This allows your friend to share details she feels comfortable sharing at that moment, whether it's a deep fear she's struggling with or what she had for lunch. Regardless of what she chooses to share, listen attentively and compassionately. And follow up later with a text saying that you've been praying for her about what she shared, so that she will feel heard and understood. When you move beyond "How are you today?" to ask other questions, remember the guidelines we discussed in chapter 4. Ask questions that show concern, seek understanding, and are appropriate for your friendship.

Include her!

Low-key social interactions can provide much-needed encouragement when your friend is feeling isolated. But she is probably not getting as many invitations as she used to, because others assume that she won't be able to join in. Continue inviting her whenever you normally would, even if you suspect that she won't be able to make it. She will be glad to be invited and to be free to make the decision herself.

If her health struggles prevent her from participating in her previous social routine, look for new ways to spend time together. This may require some creativity on your part. If you and your friend enjoyed jogging together, find a new shared activity. Call to ask if you can stop by with a snack or if she'd like to ride with you while you're running errands. Offer to bring over popcorn and a movie to watch together. Even if she needs to say no this time, she'll feel remembered and included.

Clarify public vs. private information.

If you are a close friend or relative, other people will ask you for information about how your friend is doing. This can put you in a tricky situation if you're not sure what you're allowed to share. Ask your friend to clarify which information can be shared with others and what needs to be kept private. Your friend's privacy should always trump others' desire for information. One good rule of thumb if you find yourself unprepared for these questions is to share only what your friend has shared publicly via social media or a blog. Resist the temptation to share what you know in order to impress others with your status in the inner circle. Remember, this is not about you.

Communicate others' love and concern for her.

While keeping your mouth shut is the best strategy when others want information about your friend, the opposite applies to communicating to your friend that others are thinking about her. So let your friend know when people ask you how she's doing. Remember that cancer treatment can be lonely and isolating. Sometimes it feels like the rest of the world is going on without you while you're stuck in cancer world. It helps to know that people are thinking about you and care enough to ask your friends how you're doing.

Give thoughtful gifts.

Giving gifts is another way to show love to your friend. Be sure to know your friend's situation and what she needs. If she isn't receiving chemo that causes hair loss, she doesn't need a hat! And many oncologists recommend that chemo patients avoid manicures and pedicures due to the risk of infection, so a spa gift card might not be the best choice.

The most meaningful gifts let your friend know that you're aware of her feelings and circumstances. For example, nothing says "I love you" like a large package of paper plates, napkins, cups, and utensils! To someone with no energy to do dishes and possibly with limited finances, disposable products are a blessing.

Other thoughtful gifts to consider include

- a luxurious blanket for her to carry to treatments. (Hospitals and doctors' offices can be chilly—especially if you're bald!)
- a pretty notebook for recording information at medical appointments.
- if her treatment is causing hair loss, a simple knit hat for sleeping, a chic hat for wearing out, a beautiful scarf, or high-end makeup products that will make it look like she has eyelashes and eyebrows, along with instructions for how to apply them. (If she applies heavy black eyeliner, no one will notice that she doesn't have lashes. I promise it works!)
- restaurant gift cards for meals or small gift cards for coffee, ice cream, or smoothies.
- comfortable pajamas or a new robe. (Buy button-down tops if your friend is having a mastectomy.)
- a small piece of jewelry that reminds you of your friend.
- personalized stationery for writing thank-you notes.
- an e-reader and a gift card for books. (This is a fantastic idea for a group gift—it is much easier to carry than a stack of books!)

Any small, thoughtful gift will brighten your friend's day and let her know that you care. Recruit friends, pool your resources, and surprise your friend with special gifts to encourage her throughout her journey.

This chapter may feel impossible to implement. How in the world do you provide this type of emotional support to someone who's grieving, fearful, and overwhelmed by a cancer diagnosis? You've taken a wonderful first step: taking the time to understand the emotional challenges your friend may face. In the following chapters, we'll talk more about guiding your friend through the emotional minefields she's facing and about providing spiritual support.

Questions for Reflection

1. Which of the emotions we discussed do you see your friend having? Is she typically prone to depression, anxiety, or isolation that might be worsened by her current trial?

2. How do you think your friend would respond to the "This sucks, God is good, I love you" framework of support? How can you put it into practice as you communicate with her this week?

3. Which of the gestures mentioned in this chapter would feel supportive to your friend? What do you need to do to put some of these ideas into action?

ACTION STEPS TO CONSIDER

☐ Be aware of the range of difficult, intense emotions your friend is experiencing: grief, anxiety, isolation, and feeling overwhelmed.

☐ Remember that cancer doesn't define her, and continue to talk with her about other aspects of her life and personality.

☐ Say, "This sucks, but God is good, and I love you." Acknowledge her hard circumstances, remind her of the truth of God's care for her, and show her how deeply you care.

☐ Love her by listening well. Don't worry if you say the wrong thing—nothing you can say will fix this. Ask questions, listen, and provide support, even if it's imperfect support.

☐ Love her by letting your friendship be one-sided. Don't expect her to support you emotionally. Vent to another trustworthy person when you're upset.

☐ Love her by letting her grieve. Acknowledge her fears and let her openly share them, but encourage her to stay positive and hopeful.

☐ Love her by leaving room for her questions. Be okay with not having all the answers to her struggles, and don't rush her process of wrestling through the tough questions.

☐ Love her for the long haul. Make sure she knows that you're with her for an emotional and physical marathon, not just a sprint.

- [ ] Text her often, but make sure that she knows you don't expect a response. Set an alarm to remind yourself if needed.

- [ ] Mail a card of encouragement.

- [ ] Keep up to date on how she's doing and take the time to comment on online updates.

- [ ] Instead of broadly asking, "How are you?" ask, "How are you today?" so she feels free to answer with any detail she feels comfortable sharing.

- [ ] Invite her to any social gatherings you normally would, and find new ways to enjoy each other's company if necessary.

- [ ] Give meaningful gifts that communicate concern for her feelings and circumstances.

- [ ] Read Resource 2.1: A Biblical View of Community and Resource 3.1: A Biblical View of Suffering. Their discussion of suffering and community will enrich your perspective as you support your friend emotionally.

Mind

Questions Your Friend Is Asking

I can handle the boisterous, off-key singing of "Happy Birthday" at a kid's birthday party. But, to this day, hearing a slow, solo version takes me back to 2011, a Houston living room, and my time as a bald young mom with desperate prayers for more birthdays.

I can still see the twin upholstered chairs with stacks of magazines between them, the coffee table books, and the family photos on the built-in bookshelves around the television. I spent countless hours there in the living room of my "Houston parents"—the strangers-turned-family who let me live with them during my months of treatment. When your body is wiped out from chemo and your husband and young children are six hundred miles away, there's not much to do but watch television.

So there I sat, curled up under a blanket with a knit cap covering my head and a central line coming out of my chest, watching for hours. I used to love TLC, but I had to avoid "Say Yes to the Dress" and all those moms picking out wedding dresses with their daughters, bickering, and not appreciating that they were alive to see their daughters' weddings. Cooking shows might trigger nausea. HGTV was usually safe territory.

Without fail, I'd see at least one commercial for the

American Cancer Society. That year they ran an ad campaign featuring celebrity musicians singing "Happy Birthday to You." Their tagline was "Here's to a world with more birthdays." I remember watching Celine Dion, alone on an empty concert stage, belting out her a capella rendition with emotion and heart, as my own emotions ran down my face.

I came undone each time I saw those commercials. I was diagnosed with cancer the day before my thirty-fourth birthday. I didn't expect to celebrate many more. Because of my treatment in Houston, I missed each of my children's birthdays that year. I watched them open gifts via webcam as they turned seven, five, and two.

Every single day, I begged the Lord for more birthdays. I pleaded with him to let me see my children blow out more candles, to let me live long enough for my two-year-old daughter to remember me. My idea of growing old had changed dramatically. I wasn't shooting for age seventy or eighty. In my mind, turning forty was more than I could dare to dream.

This is one of the pressing questions that cancer-fighters face: *How much time do I have left?* And it's not the only difficult question that accompanies a cancer diagnosis. You may be asking some of these troubling questions yourself. Your friend will probably struggle with these questions to varying degrees—not every cancer-fighter questions her experience and her future the same way I did. And I want to warn you that this chapter may be difficult to read, especially if you're a cancer-fighter or survivor yourself. But I think it's important to dive into these issues together. Your friend may or may not verbalize these questions, but she needs you to be aware of them, understand how they affect her, and be willing to wrestle through the answers and not give trite platitudes in response.

Why Is This Happening to Me?

In some ways, this is one question that I didn't struggle with. I knew why it was happening. I knew there was no reason that I should be exempt from the illness and death that plagues this fallen world. But I wondered about the timing and the specifics of my situation: Why couldn't I have been diagnosed when my children were old enough to remember me if I didn't survive? Why couldn't I have a more common cancer that didn't require me to travel for treatment? And I'm certain that if it had been one of my children facing cancer, I would have spent many sleepless nights asking God questions about that.

Some cancer-fighters ask this question because of dangerous, false teaching that is pervasive in the American church. Christians are being told that if you're sick, it's because of unconfessed sin in your life. God has removed his hand of protection, and the cancer swooped in. Others are told that they continue to suffer because they haven't claimed their healing by faith, as if healing were something you pick up at a coat check desk. They think, "I believe, Lord! I repent of my sin! Why is this still happening to me?" We must be prepared to help our friends navigate their questions and counter the false answers they might hear from others.

The first thing I'd say in response to the "why" question is, "We don't know." This isn't a complete answer, but it's important to acknowledge that, from a human perspective, we often can't see the reason for our suffering. We wrestle in the tension of not knowing all the answers.

The second thing I would say is that we live in a broken world plagued by sin. As we'll see in Resource 3.1, illness and death result from the fall of Adam. But we must differentiate between the consequences of sin generally and the consequences of specific sin in the life of the sick person. God sometimes uses suffering to discipline his children and punish those who reject him (see 2 Sam. 12; Heb. 12:5–11; Rev. 3:19). But, most likely, your friend's cancer is not a punishment from the Lord or a direct result of her sin.

Job 1:1 tells us that Job was righteous, and yet he suffered: "There was a man in the land of Uz whose name was Job, and that man was blameless and upright, one who feared God and turned away from evil." In John 9, Jesus and his disciples passed a man who was blind from birth. The disciples wondered out loud whether it was the man's sin or his parents' sin that had caused the affliction. "Jesus answered, 'It was not that this man sinned, or his parents, but that the works of God might be displayed in him'" (v. 3). And so we see that not all suffering is discipline or punishment for the sufferer.

Which brings us to the final part of our answer: this is happening for God's glory. We may never understand it. From our earthly perspective, we may never see God receive glory from our friend's illness. But not even cancer can prevent children of God from fulfilling their God-given purpose: to enjoy and glorify him forever.[1]

Is God Still Good?

Your friend may not ask this out loud. She may know the Sunday school answer: God is good all the time. But her feelings may be shouting a different message. God might not feel good to her in the midst of devastating circumstances. She may feel abandoned by God. What she believed before cancer about who God is may feel less true in the midst of her circumstances. You might feel the same way as you watch your friend suffer.

So let's bring these questions out into the open: Is God still good when we suffer? Yes, he is. Has he abandoned your friend? Absolutely not. Is he less faithful, less sovereign, less loving in this situation? No way. You know better than to run into your friend's struggles with your Romans 8:28 guns blazing, right? But let's ground ourselves in the truth of God's Word. He is perfectly good in all times, in all circumstances, and in all ways. He is always with us, and his character never changes. (For a deeper discussion of these topics, see Resource 3.1: A Biblical View of Suffering.)

Romans 5:8 says, "But God shows his love for us in that while we were still sinners, Christ died for us." When we look at the cross, we see God's goodness on display. On that day, he was undeniably good. He continues to show his goodness as the sun rises each morning, he provides for our needs, and he gives us good gifts.

Hebrews 13:5 tells us that God will never leave us. His presence is not dependent on our feelings. He is our God; we are his beloved children. Jesus promised his disciples that the Father would send a Helper, and now the Holy Spirit dwells in us (see John 14:26). God can't *not* be with us.

We learn in Malachi 3:6 that the Lord never changes: "For I the LORD do not change; therefore you, O children of Jacob, are not consumed." If the Lord is unchanging, his character is also unchanging. His goodness never falters. His faithfulness never wavers. His mercy and grace are poured out on his children without ceasing. Our heavenly Father is just as good to us today as he was on the day his Son died for us.

When you see your friend doubting God's goodness, presence, or character, take the time to listen to her questions and fears. Don't rush into sharing Scripture that might feel like you're judging her or dismissing her feelings. Walk with her through the valley of the shadow of death, and gently lead her to the streams of God's Word and its assurance of the Lord's unchanging goodness.

Will My Life Ever Return to Normal?

Have you ever had a terrible cold? For days, you walk around with tissues in your hand, amazed that your body could produce so much mucus. When I'm under the weather, I daydream about a day when I won't have to blow my nose. I remember having those days in the recent past—why didn't I appreciate them more?!—but it seems impossible that I will ever have one of those glorious days again. (I get a little melodramatic when I'm sick!)

When you have cancer, you feel as if life will never be normal again. I watched others care for my family and wondered if I'd ever do typical mom tasks again. I wondered if my friendships would stop being one-sided, if my energy would return, and if I'd adjust to my changed body. And those questions hurt so badly.

I remember one hard day when my friends decorated my house for Christmas. I was still in bed that morning, recovering from a chemo treatment, and my mom was at my house caring for my daughter. I heard Mom out in the living room, talking with my friends. One of my friends was taking her daughter to dance class later that morning, and they all gushed over how cute the toddler looked in her ballet outfit. I found myself unwilling to leave my bedroom and greet my friends, because I couldn't stand to see her daughter in that leotard. Instead, I stayed in my room and had a pity party. I wished that my daughter had a healthy mom who could take her to dance classes, and I wondered if I would ever do those things.

There isn't an easy answer to this question. If your friend has incurable or terminal cancer, her life will probably not return to normal. You need to prayerfully and compassionately walk alongside your friend as she navigates the grief process. We will address this unique situation in chapter 12.

If your friend has been given an encouraging prognosis, you should assure her that many aspects of her life will someday return to normal. Celebrate the milestones with her as she progresses toward the end of treatment. Keep reminding her that the end is coming. One of the most helpful comments my friend Crystal remembers from her cancer battle was when a friend told her, "One day this will be in your rearview mirror." It gave her such hope!

Yes, your friend will be forever changed by her diagnosis, physically and emotionally. Every cancer survivor I know looks back on her life and sees two distinct segments of time: B.C. (before cancer) and A.C. (after cancer). But, in many ways, her life *will* return to normal. Several months after that leotard-induced pity party, I was back to being an active mom of three. I drove school carpool, fixed slow-cooker meals, and took my daughter to a mommy-and-me music class each week. In many ways, life returned to normal, and I am still so grateful.

Am I Going to Die?

It was my nightly routine before going to bed: put on pajamas (if I'd changed out of them that day), brush my teeth, place my wig neatly on the Styrofoam head it lived on at night, and then tiptoe down the hallway to my daughter's room. I'd gently lift her out of her crib, and she'd sleepily nuzzle the shape of her slumbering body into mine, her head on my shoulder. I'd make my way to the fuzzy pink glider-rocker I had excitedly picked out when we found out we were having a girl. I would hold her, rock, weep, and pray—some nights we would rock for a few minutes, some nights for half an hour. I'd hold my baby girl and make my requests known to her heavenly Father. *Please let me live long enough for her to remember me. Please let me live long enough to walk her into first grade. Please don't let her face childhood and adolescence without her mama. Please don't let that be her story. Please, Lord.*

There's a good chance that, at some point following your friend's diagnosis, she heard or read a survival rate for her type of cancer. This little number with a percent sign after it tells you your chances of being alive five years from now. Thanks to Google, I read this number within minutes of receiving my diagnosis. I'm not sure how accurate the online information for my rare cancer was—I've seen a variety of numbers since then—but the number I read was 30 percent. In my mind, there was more than a two-thirds chance that I wouldn't be there when my baby girl started first grade. More than likely, my children would face adolescence without their mom. The odds were against me reaching middle age, and growing old felt completely unrealistic.

Cancer shatters our previously held assumptions about growing older. Even if your friend's survival chances are higher than mine were, they are probably not 100 percent. And if she's confident that she will survive, she may have been told (or may believe) that her cancer diagnosis puts her at higher risk of future cancer that could be more deadly. Let's say that she has a great prognosis with a survival rate of 80 percent. Would you want to stand in a room with ten people, knowing that two of you will be dead in five years? I wouldn't.

As a believer, my fear of death wasn't fear for myself. I long for heaven. I know that "to die is gain" (Phil. 1:21). But I was terrified for my children. I didn't want their story to be "My mom died when I was two years old . . ." I didn't want my family to suffer. I wrestled with trusting the Lord to be the good, perfect Author of their story, because it was hard to imagine any good arising from my children growing up without me.

My friend Samantha also struggled with this fear when she battled breast cancer. She said, "I knew God was there, and that he was good. But that didn't mean things would turn out the way I wanted. I knew God is good in the bad, but I really didn't want *this* bad to be his good."

Cancer also shatters our expectation of the time we will have with our loved ones. I wondered if I should be writing letters for my kids to open at their graduations and weddings or compiling a list of instructions to get my husband through his first year of single parenting. Would he know to send teacher gifts at the end of the school year? Would he remember stocking stuffers at Christmas? How would he talk to our daughter about puberty? Maybe I should be writing all this down for him!

Samantha worried that she wouldn't have time to impart all she wanted to her young children. She wanted to be there to tell them stories from her childhood and adolescence when her kids reached those ages. She found comfort in knowing that her sisters and childhood friend would fill in for her and help her kids feel like they knew her. But she still felt immense pressure to leave something for her kids. She didn't want them to wish they had more from her. I've heard this concern from numerous cancer-fighters.

When you're struggling with this fear, reminders are everywhere. I remember being jealous of elderly people. I couldn't handle hearing friends talk about raising teenagers. I didn't want to discuss retirement savings or daydream about my children's graduations or weddings. These conversations reminded me that I might not live to parent a teenager, grow old with my husband, or hold my grandbabies.

If your friend voices her concerns about death, let her talk about her feelings. I know this is a tough conversation. I struggle to go there with my friends who are battling cancer today. It makes me uncomfortable, sad, and scared. I want to be optimistic and not have those discussions, because I don't want to think about my friend dying. But we can love our friends by being a safe place for them to voice their fears.

Samantha described it this way: "You don't want to feel like you have to argue the validity of your fears. Friends feel like they need to help you think it isn't going to happen—but you already think it's going to happen. It would be better if they embraced your fears and let you talk about it. If someone doesn't go there with you easily, then you probably won't talk about it with her again. You don't want to be a downer."

Once you have listened to your friend's fears, how should you respond? Your first response should always be aimed at letting her know she's been heard. Don't dismiss her fears or say, "I know you'll be fine!" Instead, say something like "I'm so sorry you're facing this. It must be awful having to wrestle through it all. I'm willing to listen anytime."

Second, reassure her of your continued support, even if her worst fears come true. As I mentioned in chapter 8, I was encouraged when a close friend told me that she would help my husband with our kids. But you want to choose your wording carefully. Your friend needs you to have the conversation with her but also to remain hopeful for her. If your friend's cancer is curable, you might say something like "I know you're going to survive this. But if you don't, your family won't be left on their own. All of us will rally around them." Don't make promises that you aren't prepared to keep, but reassure your friend if you can.

If she's facing a terminal illness, be ready to talk about these topics, but only if she brings them up first. If the discussion arises, consider asking her if there are specific ways she wants you to support her family when she's gone. Are there stories she'd like you to share with her children? Specific roles she wants you to play in their lives as they grow? Be willing to engage in these difficult discussions with her if she asks you to.

Once you've listened and reassured her, carefully point her back to the truth about the Lord. The Author of her family's story is her loving, faithful, merciful heavenly Father. He loves her, and he loves her family. We can't understand his ways, but we can have confidence in the unchanging nature of his character. Samantha felt encouraged in her fears for her family by thinking about them in light of eternity. She knew that even if her children suffered through most of their lifetimes without her, their suffering would be temporary. We grieve the devastation of illness and death, but we do not grieve without hope.

None of these questions have easy answers. They are questions we aren't used to asking, and they may be taboo in some Christian churches. If your friend doesn't feel comfortable talking about her fears and doubts, she will feel even more isolated from others. Whether or not your friend utters any of these questions out loud, your emotional support will be more compassionate when you're sensitive to her struggles rumbling beneath the surface. And if she decides to open up about these questions, you'll be ready to listen and wrestle through these issues with her.

Questions for Reflection

1. Which of the questions in this chapter do you think your friend might be wrestling through? (If you are a close friend, you may consider asking her.)
2. How can you listen and support your friend as she processes her difficult emotions and questions?

ACTION STEPS TO CONSIDER

☐ Listen compassionately as your friend struggles through tough questions.

☐ Be aware of questions she may be wrestling with, even if she doesn't share them with you.

☐ Communicate support without using platitudes, dismissing her questions, or judging her.

Soul

Praying and Understanding Spiritual Needs

During one of the most difficult times in my treatment for cancer, my friend Sarah had a dream that she shared with me. Here is her description of the dream, in her own words:

We were in a very large, cathedral-style church. The pews were packed with people—some I recognized from church, but many I did not recognize at all. Everyone was praying and writing. They were writing their prayers. At the front of the church, the stage was some sort of hospital room, and you were lying on a table with doctors and nurses bustling around you. I talked to one woman who said, "I don't know Marissa personally, but I'm honored to be here to pray for her." I was amazed at the outpouring of prayer for you and your healing. Everyone was giving you their prayers after they wrote them down as they left the church. I peeked at some of the letters and they all began with praise to God by worshiping his Name (mighty God, everlasting Father, omniscient, all-powerful, etc., just like we've learned from Isaiah). SO AWESOME.

Her dream was an encouragement to me at a time of intense struggle and sorrow, because I knew that it accurately depicted what was happening before the throne of the almighty God. Many people were interceding on my behalf, including many I have never met. I regularly received cards from strangers saying that they were praying for me. I received dozens of small yellow postcards from the prayer room of a church in Tennessee, letting me know that someone had prayed for me. I still don't know who put my name on that prayer list, but I'm thankful.

Nothing is as powerful as bringing your friend before the throne of her Creator and Redeemer. Interceding on her behalf before the Lord of the universe is one of the greatest gifts you can give her. Long after the doctors tell her that she's cancer-free, keep your friend on your list for frequent prayer. And if the Lord calls your friend home to heaven, keep fervently praying for her loved ones.

Why You Should Pray

If you've stayed with me through nine chapters, I probably don't need to convince you to pray for your friend. But here are two reasons I encourage you to do so:

1. Your friend needs you to pray.

In Exodus 17, the Israelites battled Amalek in the wilderness. As Joshua led the people into battle, Moses stood on a hill with Aaron and Hur and held the staff of God. When Moses's hands were in the air, the Israelites were winning. But when his hands grew weary and dropped to his side, the people of Amalek gained ground. As the battle dragged on, Moses sat on a rock, and Aaron and Hur held up his arms. And so the Israelites defeated Amalek.

Your friend needs you to be her Aaron and Hur as her arms tire. Your friend may struggle to pray when she's in pain, exhausted, foggy from chemo, discouraged, or entrenched in survival mode. You can stand in the gap and pray for her.

When Anna's mother was diagnosed with stage four breast cancer, it felt like her world was falling apart. Anna told a friend, "I can't pray and talk to a God who would let this happen." Her friend replied, "Then I'll pray for you." Whether your friend admits her prayer struggles to you or not, you have an opportunity to go before the Lord on her behalf. Don't waste it. She needs you.

2. You need to pray.

I know that you're worried about your friend. You're sad and hurting, too. And Scripture is clear about the best response to our troubles. Philippians 4:6–7 gives a command and a promise: "Do not be anxious about anything, but in everything by prayer and supplication with thanksgiving let your requests be made known to God. And the peace of God, which surpasses all understanding, will guard your hearts and your minds in Christ Jesus." First Peter 5:7 says, "Cast all your anxiety on him because he cares for you" (NIV). God's Word teaches us to bring our pain and our worries to him.

When you're scared for your friend, the best response is prayer. Come to the throne of grace and receive mercy and comfort (see Heb. 4:16). When we pray, we acknowledge that we need the Lord. We don't have all the answers, but he is perfect wisdom and strength. We bend our hearts to his sovereign will, and he meets us in our pain with his guidance, comfort, and peace. Run to him in prayer, and you will find what you need.

How to Pray for Your Friend

Pray for healing for your friend, of course. But don't stop there. Here are some additional ways to pray for your friend.

- Pray for her to feel the closeness of the Lord as he strengthens, sustains, and comforts her (see Pss. 62:1–2; 63:5–8; Isa. 41:10).
- Pray for wisdom for her friends and family members so they can support and encourage her in ways that she needs the most (James 1:5).
- Pray against her feelings of isolation—physically, emotionally, and spiritually (Josh. 1:9; Pss. 42; 56:8; Heb. 13:5).
- Pray for wisdom in making medical decisions so that your friend, her family members, and the doctors will not have any regrets (Ps. 112:7–8).
- If she's married, pray that God will strengthen her marriage and deepen her connection with her husband, and that she will look to the Lord to meet her needs when her husband falls short (Eph. 5:22–23).
- Pray that she would develop a deep and abiding trust in the Lord and will not place her hope in a particular outcome but wholly in God's character: his sovereignty, goodness, and faithfulness to her specifically in this situation (Isa. 43; Jer. 31:3; Rom. 8:38–39).
- Pray that she will feel free to ask for help and support when she needs it, claiming the promise that God will meet all her needs according to his glorious riches in Christ Jesus (Phil. 4:19).
- Pray for her to feel joy and peace, as she grieves the loss of her health and her "before cancer" expectations for her life, and not to be anxious about the future (Lam. 3:21–24; Rom. 15:13; Phil. 4:6–8).
- Pray that she will not waste her suffering but will be transformed and sanctified through the experience of suffering for God's glory (Rom. 8:28–29; 12:1–2).
- Pray that God will prepare her to comfort others with the comfort that she is now receiving (2 Cor. 1:3–4).

These are all important ways to pray for your friend, but be careful when you pray *with* your friend. In the past, I've been guilty of using prayer to remind friends of truths that I think they've forgotten. The prayer ends up sounding like a sermon. We've all heard (or prayed) the sermon-prayers: "Dear Lord, please help Katie to trust that you work all things together for her good . . ." As we discussed in chapter 4, we need to be careful with our religious platitudes in prayer as well.

Meeting Other Spiritual Needs

Prayer is not your friend's only spiritual need. Having a biblical view of suffering is equally important, so that she can discern truth in the various statements she will hear from others about her suffering. (See Resource 3.1 for more on a biblical view of suffering.) And don't forget biblically based comfort and encouragement that will offer her something more than the ephemeral ideas or empty platitudes that people may offer. Give her something to hold on to—truth offers a strong, stable grounding.

Your friend needs a biblical view of suffering.

During my illness, and for years following it, I spent a great deal of time thinking about suffering. When I was diagnosed, I was grateful to have a well-stocked spiritual pantry. I knew the truth about the Lord's character, but I needed more. As I walked through suffering, my experience drove me deeper into God's Word as I searched for understanding.

This perspective doesn't develop overnight. I haven't arrived at a perfect or complete understanding of the topic, but it's been helpful to me to grow in my understanding of what God's Word says about suffering. I need to sort the truth from the lies as I talk to others and hear messages in the world and in the church. You and your friend need to do this, too. You can help both of you to develop a biblical view of suffering by knowing what God's Word says about suffering.

First, spend time studying what God's Word says about suffering and how God walks with us through pain and trials. When I was sick, a friend shared with me a sermon series from the book of Job. I shared it with two of my best friends, and they listened to it as well. It provided a springboard for excellent discussions that encouraged and strengthened us.

Ask your friend if any verses, sermons, or books encourage her, and join her in learning from them. Read what she's reading and listen to what she's listening to. Or find resources that the two of you can explore together. Some of my favorite books about suffering are listed in the For Further Reading section at the back of this book. Joni Eareckson Tada's book, *A Place of Healing*, is a great place to start.

Listen for clues to discern what your friend is believing or hearing about her suffering. Even well-meaning Christians often tell suffering people things that are not true. She may be told that her illness is due to unconfessed sin in her life. She might hear that if she has unwavering faith, she will be healed. And she will probably hear, at least once, "God will never give you more than you can handle." None of these statements are biblical, so equip yourself with the knowledge of God's Word so that you can help her sort through people's words and proclaim God's truth. We saw in chapter 9 that the stories of Job and Jesus healing the man who was born blind teach us that suffering is not always due to the sin of the suffering person (see Job 1 and John 9). God's sovereignty throughout the Bible shows us that he does as he wills, and his plans do not depend on our good faith or behavior. The phrase "God will never give you more than you can handle" is not in the Bible.[1] If we believe this to be one of God's promises and then see that we've been given more difficulty than we can handle on our own, we may doubt whether any of God's promises are true. The truth is that God *will* give us more than we alone can bear—and, when he does, he teaches us to rely solely on him.

Your friend needs biblical comfort.

We've talked throughout this book about your friend's need for your compassion and comfort. When we consider sadness in the context of God's Word, we see our friend's tears not as a weakness to be rebuked but as a call for us to surround her with God's comfort. Her tears do not indicate a lack of faith. Psalm 56:8 tells us that our heavenly Father keeps a record of our tears. He cares about our sadness, and he cares for us in our sadness.

In the Sermon on the Mount, Jesus said, "Blessed are those who mourn, for they shall be comforted" (Matt. 5:4). Jesus doesn't shun those who mourn or tell them to hurry up with their grieving. He promises comfort, and you are one way that he comforts your grieving friend. When Jesus returns, he isn't coming only to judge the world and establish his reign on earth. He is coming to wipe away every tear from our eyes. You can use these truths about the Lord to comfort your friend in her sadness.

Your friend needs biblical encouragement.

When you know what Scripture says about God's character and promises, you can comfort your friend with his Word during dark days of despair or hopelessness. But do this gently. Remember our discussion about religious platitudes in chapter 4? When your friend is hurting, take time to sit with her in her pain. Don't give flippant answers.

As you grieve with her, gently and lovingly point her to the One who heals all her diseases—the physical, emotional, and spiritual. Turn her eyes to the One who loves her, strengthens her, and will never leave her (see Jer. 31:3, Phil. 4:13, Heb. 13:5). Constantly remind her of the truth about her Redeemer and his promises. This is not easy to navigate. But God promises to be with us and give us wisdom (see Isa. 30:21, James 1:5).

Let's talk about practical steps you can take to encourage your friend spiritually. In my experience, my spiritual health was strengthened when friends reminded me of Scripture and let me know that they were praying for me. Thankfully, the texts, emails, and cards never stopped. One friend sent emails to everyone who had accessed my CaringBridge blog and asked them to send me index cards with Scripture on them. Organizing a similar "Scripture shower" would be a wonderful way to encourage your friend spiritually. Spread the word, and buy her a pretty box or another way to store the cards she receives.

Brainstorm ways to keep Scripture in front of your friend. Consider buying her a cute chalkboard or dry-erase board and, whenever you're in her home, write a Bible verse on it. On days when you know she is struggling, set alarms at intervals during the day. When the alarm goes off, pray for your friend and text her an encouraging verse. (See Resource 4.1 for suggestions of verses to comfort your friend.)

On my darkest days, when I couldn't fathom how I could keep going, a well-timed note or text would bring the encouragement I needed. My community was not just the hands and feet of Christ, doing what needed to be done—they were the heart and arms of Christ, meeting my spiritual needs and comforting me along the way.

Questions for Reflection

1. Which of the ways to pray for your friend were new or thought provoking for you?

2. What obstacles are standing in the way of you regularly praying for your friend? If you have a hard time remembering to pray, would periodic alarms or calendar reminders help you to consistently pray?
3. How could you set aside specific time to pray for your friend? Who else could you ask to pray with you?
4. In what ways do you see your friend wrestling spiritually? What biblical truth could be beneficial to her in her struggle?
5. What are some ways that you could keep God's promises in front of your friend?

ACTION STEPS TO CONSIDER

☐ Pray for your friend regularly (and set alarms to help you remember). You can use the resource on page 251 to keep track of your friend's prayer requests and your prayers for her.

☐ Tell her (through texts, emails, etc.) when you pray for her—the knowledge of your prayers will encourage and nourish her spiritually.

☐ Study what God's Word says about suffering so that you can counter lies your friend might hear about God and cancer. Read Resource 3.1: A Biblical View of Suffering and then see the For Further Reading section at the back of this book for other book suggestions.

☐ Do not shy away from your friend's tears; instead, meet her tears with comfort from God's Word.

☐ Encourage your friend with Scripture. Consider organizing a "Scripture shower" by asking others to mail her index cards with Scriptures, buying her a dry-erase board and keeping it filled with verses, or texting her regularly—whatever you can do to keep God's promises in the forefront of her mind.

When Her Husband, Parent, or Child Has Cancer

Supporting a Friend as She Cares for Others

We've spent ten chapters discussing how to love your friend through cancer. But what if your friend doesn't have cancer? What if the disease has struck her spouse, parent, or child? If that's the case, then this chapter is for you. If you've turned here first, welcome! This is a great place to start. This chapter will highlight the unique characteristics of your friend's situation and how you can help. I hope that you'll read the rest of the book as well. As I've talked to friends whose husbands, parents, and children had cancer, I've discovered that their needs were similar to those of us who had cancer ourselves. You'll find their stories here, as well as woven into many of this book's chapters.

When a Friend's Husband Has Cancer

When Lisa's husband was diagnosed with leukemia, she watched as family and friends packed themselves into his hospital room. The road ahead was still plagued by uncertainty, but one thing she knew was that it wouldn't be easy. Over the months that followed, her husband's health plodded slowly toward remission, and an inner circle of family and friends stepped up to serve them consistently and compassionately. I'm thankful for her willingness, and the willingness of other wives who have walked this road, to share what helped them feel loved during that difficult time.

Bring meals.

When a friend's husband is ill, we may assume that she can handle her normal responsibilities. We need to consider the impact of her husband's illness on her time, energy, and capacity for doing other tasks. When Lisa's husband was sick, there were many days when caring for her husband and taking him to treatment consumed her time. She was healthy and able to cook, but she felt loved when friends provided meals on her husband's long treatment days.

Be aware of your friend's husband's medical situation, his treatment schedule, and when meals could be helpful. Even if she insists that meals aren't necessary, you could stock her freezer with meals to lighten her load.

Give the caregiver a break.

Her husband's illness means increased stress and responsibility for your friend. Consider how her daily life has changed and how you can help to carry her burden. She may suddenly shoulder responsibility for tasks like paying bills, handling finances, dealing with insurance issues, caring for the lawn, getting the cars serviced, and handling household and parenting responsibilities alone. She may be driving her husband to appointments and caring for him after surgery or chemo. She's not sick, but cancer is affecting her daily life. She needs your tangible support.

When surgery or inpatient treatment requires a hospital stay, your friend might be eager to run errands, head home to take a shower, or have a few hours of normalcy. During times when the medical situation isn't critical but her husband still needs someone with him, you or your husband could give her a break by staying with her husband for awhile. Be sure to bring a book so that he knows he doesn't need to entertain you if he doesn't feel well. And don't force the issue if your friend doesn't want to leave his side. But consider asking, "Would you like me to pick up groceries for you? Or would you rather I come sit with him while you get out?"

Your friend would probably love a girls' night out or a lunch with friends to take her mind off her troubles for a while. You could recruit someone to stay with her husband while you whisk her way for a few hours. If they have small children at home, time alone together would be a wonderful gift to give your friend and her husband. Take the children with you so the adults have the option of staying home if there are emotional discussions that need to happen without little ears overhearing.

Be sensitive to her fears.

We've talked about the anxiety that cancer patients face, and spouses face many of those same fears. When I was walking through cancer, I was aware that, if it didn't end well, I'd be dancing with Jesus while my husband would be left to raise grieving children. I didn't fear death in the same way that my husband feared my death. When our friend's husband faces cancer, we need to be sympathetic to the emotions she's working through as she considers the possibility of being the one left behind.

When Liz's husband faced major cancer surgery, the risk was high, and she was frightened. They had two young boys, and she faced possible widowhood as she looked at the operation's success rate. She was comforted when a friend reminded her that her husband wasn't a statistic. This friend didn't ignore or dismiss Liz's fears, but she gently spoke words of truth and encouragement. (And Liz's husband came through the risky surgery with no evidence of cancer afterward!)

It's important not to be flippant in your response to her fears, but try not to be pessimistic, either. Recognize her fear, meet her in her pain, and let her know that she's not alone. Remember what we talked about in chapter 8: repeatedly communicate your support, but don't expect her to respond.

When a Friend's Parent Has Cancer

My friend Anna and I sat in brown leather chairs in the middle of Starbucks, gripping our lattes and leaning in close as her young daughter ran circles around us. Days earlier, Anna's mom had been diagnosed with stage four breast cancer—a recurrence after more than a decade of good health. I invited Anna out for coffee to hear how she was handling the news. I listened as she told me with tears in her eyes that she never expected this. Even after her mom's first battle with cancer, she never let herself think it could come back. She told me, "This news would hit me like a truck even if I thought I'd prepared myself for it. I'm thankful that I didn't waste her healthy years worrying." In those emotional moments, Anna needed someone outside her family to understand how difficult her mother's diagnosis was. She needed more than a text reply with a couple of crying emojis and hearts. She needed friends to show up, listen to her sorrow, and walk with her through the painful years that followed.

Acknowledge the hard.

Our friends need us to understand the pain caused by a parent's illness, even when we ourselves are adults. When Ashley's mom battled stage four breast cancer, she faced not only losing her mom, but losing a best friend and the grandmother of her newborn and three-year-old daughters. Her mom played more than one significant role in their family's life, and she grieved each one as its own loss. She needed to know that her friends were brokenhearted with her and loved her mom, too.

When some friends spoke to Ashley with clichés such as "God's in control" or "Everything will work out," she felt like they didn't understand how distressing the situation was. She told me, "When they acted like it was no big deal, that wasn't helpful. I needed my friends to acknowledge that it was hard and to be on their knees for my mom."

Don't forget to ask your friend regularly how she and her parent are doing. If her cancer-fighting parent doesn't live locally, the illness may not affect her life on a daily basis, but it certainly affects her emotions. Make sure your friend knows that you remember what she's going through and are praying for her family.

Free her to be present with her parent.

When we're busy with our own families, it's difficult for us to help our aging parents—especially those who are receiving cancer treatment. I spoke with multiple friends whose mothers battled breast cancer, and they all told me it was important for them to join their moms at chemotherapy appointments. But they all had young children and hectic households. They desperately wanted that time with their moms, but it was difficult to work out the logistics.

You can love your friend by keeping her kids or lightening her responsibilities at home by cleaning, bringing meals, or helping with errands. This will free her to spend the time she needs with her mom. She also carries an emotional burden, and watching her mom receive chemo is hard. If you can keep the kids during the appointment and also offer a little extra time for her to emotionally process and decompress, that will be especially helpful.

During Alexis's mom's prolonged battle with breast cancer, she spent a lot of time at her parents' house. She spent hours every week driving to their house, cooking for them, and serving them. It was stressful for her to keep up her own responsibilities at home, so anything that friends could take off her plate was helpful. During Anna's mom's illness, she drove to their home in a nearby town often, and gas cards were a blessing. She also appreciated restaurant gift cards that she could use to feed not only her family but her parents as well. A friend brought her dinner once a week, and this allowed her to spend extra time with her parents on those days.

You can also free her to be present with her parent by lowering the expectations for your friendship. Alexis told me that she didn't have time to give to other people when her mom was sick. She wanted to tell her friends, "Your friendship will be here later. Right now, I need to focus on my mom."

Understand her changed role.

While her parent is sick, or if she loses her parent, your friend may assume new roles in her extended family. She may care for an ill mother or a caregiving father. She may spend extra time with a surviving parent who loses their spouse. She may organize holiday gatherings that used to be hosted by her parents. These changes are difficult to navigate, especially when they are emotionally complicated by illness and/or loss. Take the time to ask your friend how her parent's illness is affecting her, and listen compassionately. This difficult situation is probably affecting more than just her weekly schedule, and she'll appreciate your sensitivity to her new reality.

If she loses her parent to cancer, remember that birthdays and holidays can be especially difficult. Ask your friend which holidays are most painful—it could be Christmas, Mother's or Father's Day, her parent's birthday, or even her own birthday. Mark your calendar and recognize these difficult dates with a card, flowers, or a meal for her family as she's grieving, and continue to do so even after the first year.

When a Friend's Child Has Cancer

Neither of us belonged at the small playground in a posh Houston neighborhood. We were both transplanted there against our will for the sake of cancer treatment at the hospitals that were blocks away. While I was at MD Anderson Cancer Center, this young mother spent time roaming the halls of Texas Children's Hospital, praying for a cure for her daughter's leukemia. We watched her two daughters play and talked about the effects of cancer on our families, marriages, checkbooks, and hearts. I realized that this young mom faced all the same fears I did but also bore many additional burdens. I was able to keep life mostly normal for the rest of my family; their entire crew had moved to Houston. I had hours in bed to process my emotions; she was still caring for her family and parenting two children, one of whom was battling for her life. I wondered how my children would cope if I didn't survive; she faced the possibility of living the rest of her life without her child.

Understand their unique situation.

Not every case of childhood cancer is the same, but there are challenges that are common to many. Most childhood cancers require aggressive treatment and lengthy hospital stays. Treatment often begins immediately or just days after diagnosis. It usually occurs at children's hospitals, requiring families to travel, or even relocate, to hospitals in another city or

state for months or years. And there is one common denomi-
nator for all parents of childhood cancer patients: the battle is
all-consuming.

Parents watch their child suffer, knowing that if they survive, there will be long-lasting implications. Treatment is often
risky, and parents are faced with difficult choices. They may be
required to sacrifice aspects of their child's long-term health,
choosing infertility, organ damage, and other permanent side
effects in an effort to save the child's life. When you talk with
your friend, be satisfied with what she's willing to share. She
and her husband may need time to process all that's happening
and the constant ups and downs before they're ready to share
details with others.

Friendships are quickly formed within the childhood cancer community. Women befriend other women who are qui-
etly weeping in hospital restrooms. They walk the dark road
of uncertainty and pain together. Parents of survivors watch
other children relapse or pass away, exacerbating their own
fear and sadness. It's a precious community but also a difficult
one. Listen patiently if your friend confides in you about these
new friendships, and don't feel threatened by them. She needs
you to understand both the importance of her community and
the emotional toll that it sometimes takes.

When Courtney's three-year-old daughter battled a stage
4 Wilm's tumor, she knew that their normal wasn't normal to
other people around them. She needed friends to understand
how unpredictable their days were. She never knew when her
daughter might be admitted to the hospital. Courtney couldn't
plan social events. She didn't accept invitations often, but she
wanted her friends to continue pursuing her. She needed
friends to be patient and to understand that their family life
was going to revolve around cancer for a long time.

Keep in mind that not every childhood cancer comes with

lengthy treatment and a poor prognosis. When the diagnosis comes, give the family time to learn the next steps and communicate their needs. When Aimee's teenage son was diagnosed with lymphoma, friends assumed that they faced lengthy, out-of-town treatment. Aimee received phone calls from distraught friends and many monetary gifts and gift cards. As they received results from further diagnostic testing, her son's prognosis was excellent and didn't require chemotherapy. She felt guilty that they had received so many gifts and didn't need them. She wishes that people had waited until they had more information before jumping to conclusions.

Support their marriage.

Childhood cancer is rough on a marriage. Some families are physically separated when one parent travels with the child for treatment or spends nights at the hospital and another parent stays home to work and/or care for their other children. This arrangement may go on for months or even years. The stress of watching your child suffer and the fear of losing her, along with financial and logistical struggles, can further strain a marriage. When Courtney's daughter was hospitalized for long periods of time, there were weeks when she and her husband saw each other only as they passed in the hospital hallway. She recommends that friends offer to stay with the child while the parents spend time together, even if it's just a quick stroll on the hospital lawn.

Remember that they're facing enormous stress and may not be able to step away from the hospital for long. When Jess's infant daughter was hospitalized, Jess and her husband left her side one evening for a rare, quick dinner together. While they were gone, her mother-in-law called to tell them that their daughter had been placed on a ventilator, and they rushed back. They felt like they could never take a break. Keep offering to give your friend and her husband time alone together, but remember that she may not feel like she can get away. You may need to find other ways to surround their marriage with your prayer and support.

Meet tangible needs.

Your friend's needs will depend on her specific circumstances, but here are some ideas from parents who have been there. They suggest sending gifts when a family is facing a long hospitalization: toys, games, books, or puzzles for the hospitalized child; snacks and paper goods; ibuprofen; and soft Kleenex. When Courtney's daughter was diagnosed, they were given a large binder containing applications for numerous assistance programs for families. But her life was too busy and stressful to navigate many of these programs. She recommends asking your friend if there are resources you could research and apply for on their behalf.

If the family is away from home for long periods of time, gather friends to help maintain their yard, collect their mail, pay bills, and care for other needs around the house. You could also ease their homesickness by texting photos or sending care packages with reminders of home. They may enjoy small gift cards that could be used for a special treat. Remember, the best gifts don't require anything from the family. Organize a fundraiser, but don't expect the family to make an appearance. Send an anonymous gift that doesn't need a thank-you note. Your friend will appreciate your one-sided, practical support of her family.

Keep showing up.

Your persistent presence lets them know that they're not forgotten. But when you visit, leave your expectations behind. When Jess's daughter was hospitalized, they spent most of their time in the pediatric intensive care unit. If they wanted to greet visitors, they needed to leave the PICU and head out to the waiting room. Many times, they couldn't or didn't want to step away from their daughter. You can encourage your friend by letting her know that your presence doesn't come with conditions. Jess recommends leaving a card or a small treat so that the parents know you were there, but be okay with not seeing them face-to-face.

Pam's three-year-old son's battle with stage 4, high-risk neuroblastoma spanned four years of ups and downs, various treatments, and clinical trials in multiple states. She told me, "I wasn't able to respond or be a good friend back for a long time. I wish that more friends had taken the initiative and asked me to go for a walk or out for coffee, rather than being scared on the sidelines." She needed friends who were comfortable with her tears and were willing to keep reaching out even when she didn't have anything to give in return. Whether it's your friend, her husband, her parent, or her child who's facing cancer, you can bless her by being this kind of friend: relentlessly pursuing, loving, praying, and serving, for as long as it takes, with no expectation of your efforts being reciprocated.

When I met Lisa for coffee on a sunny Sunday afternoon to interview her for this chapter, she texted me to let me know she was running late. She'd gotten a flat tire and was waiting for her husband to drive out and help her change it. When she arrived for our interview, we chatted about how his cancer battle years earlier had changed her perspective. Getting a flat tire was an annoyance, but she was thankful to have a healthy husband to help her. She knows not to take this for granted. Whether your friend's loved one survives or receives eternal healing with the Lord, she will be changed by the experience. It's difficult to be the one who's sick and considering your mortality, but it's also tough to be the one who might be left behind to grieve. As you pray for her, serve her, and love her well, you can also point her to Christ. He is her unchanging, steadfast Rock of refuge when nothing else feels the same.

Questions for Reflection

1. What did you learn from this chapter about the unique nature of your friend's situation?
2. How can you tailor your support based on the practical advice that was given in this chapter?

ACTION STEPS TO CONSIDER

☐ When a friend's husband has cancer, bring meals to lighten her load, make sure she gets a break, and acknowledge her fears with compassion.

☐ When a friend's parent has cancer, recognize her painful circumstances, help her with childcare or other responsibilities so she can spend time with her ailing parent, and understand her changed family roles.

☐ When a friend's child has cancer, understand their unique situation, support their marriage, meet their tangible needs, and keep showing up.

When There's No Cure

Supporting a Friend through Chronic or Terminal Illness

We sat on her deck with the takeout I brought for lunch, chatting while we inhaled the shimmering lake and blue sky. Jean didn't eat much, which concerned me. An oxygen tank sat nearby, ignored by its beneficiary because of my presence. She hated for others to see her weakness. She was used to being strong. She was a fighter, a feisty competitor, full of energy, enthusiasm, and spunk. But now the strength was slipping away.

We were diagnosed with cancer on the same day—my favorite high school teacher and me. Angiosarcoma for me, stage 4 breast cancer for her—and neither of us likely to survive five years. And yet, here we were, five years later. Both of us were finished with treatment, but for different reasons.

When Jean retired from her work and started several months of in-home hospice care, I went to visit. She kept asking me to come back, and, as my visits grew more regular, our friendship deepened. At first, I didn't think I could do it. I didn't think I could watch her deteriorate. I didn't think I could handle her slow march toward heaven. But I also couldn't abandon our friendship just because it was hard.

We spent the first couple of visits mostly sharing memories

and catching up. As time went on, our visits were less about two people who shared a past and more about two people who were sharing the present. But looming over our friendship was the unavoidable fact that one of us faced a short future. We talked about family, faith, fear, cancer, and dying.

And now she is gone, taken home to glory, finally healed. Jean wasn't the first friend I lost to cancer, and she probably won't be the last. Cancer in all forms is devastating, but the pain of knowing that a friend won't be healed in this life is excruciating.

If your friend has been diagnosed with incurable cancer, I am deeply sorry. This is difficult to talk about, but it's important to address the unique challenges of incurable patients. Even without a cure, your friend could have several years of life ahead of her. Her journey will look considerably different from a short-term illness that lasts a few months and results in a complete remission. It may be a marathon, filled with ups and downs and challenging emotions.

Unique Challenges

I spoke with several friends as I prepared to write this chapter, and the common theme that ran through their comments was this: "Please don't forget about me and what I'm going through." In a long-term illness, the support that your friend experiences in the beginning can fade as people grow weary, move on to other crises, become discouraged by negative medical developments, or grow fearful of her last days. Your friend may be looking around at her circle of friends, wondering, *Who will stick around? Who can handle walking through this with me?*

Your friend knows that people don't know what to say. She understands that her presence sometimes makes others feel awkward. She sees people dodge her in the school pickup line or the grocery store. And while it hurts when she's treated this way by acquaintances, her real fear is that her friends will pull away and abandon her in her time of greatest need.

Incurable patients often endure several attempts at treatment—some successful, some unsuccessful—and so their journeys involve frequent ups and downs. Treatment may keep the cancer at bay for a while, only for it to return months later. Your friend may be in the unenviable position of having to communicate disappointing or devastating news to those around her. She'll appreciate people who are steadfast through the highs and lows.

Your friend needs you to acknowledge the struggle she's going through and to value her experience enough to enter into her pain. She'll feel loved when you stay updated on what's happening. There's a battle going on in her mind—a battle to stay hopeful so she can fully live each day she is given while knowing that her days are numbered. Hearing from those who are thinking of her or praying for her will strengthen her.

Your friend probably has a high need for contact and support, coupled with a low capacity for responding to that contact. Her energy—both physically and emotionally—will be limited much of the time. Send text messages and emails that don't require a response, leave a meal in a cooler on the front porch, or ship a gift that surprises her in the mail. These are meaningful ways to let her know that you care without requiring a lot of effort on her part to engage. Try to maximize your expression of support and minimize her need to respond to it.

If you send a card, avoid those that say "Get well soon" or "Best wishes on the road to recovery." These phrases insult someone with a terminal illness, and your card will make her feel misunderstood rather than supported. Instead, select a "Thinking of you" card, and write a personalized message inside.

I know that you're hurting, too, as you prepare to say goodbye. This is so hard. You're probably walking through uncharted territory while grieving and pouring yourself out for your friend. You need support, too. But, as we've discussed in previous chapters, your friend who is sick will not provide that support for you. Remember, only communicate support to her—and vent to others outside her inner circle while being careful to avoid gossip. Find a trustworthy friend, a pastor, or a counselor who can listen as you process your emotions.

Matching Your Friend's Tone

When I'm relating to a friend in this situation, I often struggle with what to say. Should I be optimistic and hopeful? Does she need me to acknowledge her medical prognosis and join in any fear or sadness that she's currently feeling? I've walked through chronic and terminal illness with friends and have seen their various needs. Not only will one person's needs vary wildly from another friend's—the same friend may herself have different needs from one hour to the next. I've decided the best approach is to match your friend's tone from moment to moment.

When my friend Jamie's husband first received a diagnosis of incurable, stage four colon cancer, they needed friends to understand the reality of his prognosis. They didn't need people to tell them stories of a friend who had colon cancer at an earlier stage and was cured. They needed to grieve and emotionally process what they were facing.

Yet, when they started chemo treatment and the ups and downs of fighting the cancer—fighting for more time and praying for a miracle—they needed to feel hopeful. If they dwelled on the medical statistics, they wouldn't have the energy for the fight. During that phase, they needed friends to be upbeat and to join them in praying for the best outcome possible.

When it was clear that her husband would not be healed on earth, Jamie and her husband longed for love and support. They needed those in their inner circle to keep pursuing them, even if they didn't respond. And they needed friends in the outer circles to keep praying and communicating support—again, without needing or expecting a response.

Your friend's attitude and need for emotional support will shift many times during her journey through her illness. Keep asking questions and try to match how she's feeling each day as you communicate support. If she's grieving, grieve with her. If she's fighting, put on your fighting gloves and communicate hope and encouragement. And, when the end draws near, keep letting her know that you're still with her, that you love her, and that you will never, ever forget her.

Logistical Issues

At some point, your friend and her family will probably transition from crisis mode to a "new normal" way of life. She knows that people are busy, and she doesn't expect her supporters to maintain the same intensity of involvement you would expect in a short-term illness. But she still needs help and support from her friends.

Years of treatment take a toll on your friend's body. Even when she's feeling her best, she may not have the energy to run errands, do housework, or tackle big projects like cleaning out closets. Keep offering to help with these things. When you do something at your house, such as cleaning out your kid's closet at the end of the season, remember that this might not have happened at her house in years. There may be times when she can't drive because of medications. You can offer to chauffeur her to appointments, to work, or to run errands. This act of service has the added benefit of giving you some time with your friend! And if she has kids, they probably have transportation needs as well. Even if your friend doesn't take you up on your offers of help, they serve as a reminder that you're still aware of her situation and are right there, willing and able to support her.

When these logistical needs go on for several years, it might work well to assign friends to specific days of the week. On your assigned day, you are responsible for anything that your friend and her family needs that day—transporting kids, picking up groceries, and other logistical tasks. This way, several friends can share the responsibilities without one person feeling overwhelmed.

If you provide help with her children, respect her style of parenting and mirror it as much as possible. This includes the difficult task of providing consistent structure and discipline. It's tempting to want to coddle the kids or compensate for the hardship in their family by making every day into a party. But, in a long-term situation, treating the kids differently can make them feel pitied and cause major problems down the road. While you will likely want to spoil your friend's kids, you can help her (and them!) more by having the same expectations for her kids as you would for your own.

Don't Let Her Become Invisible

In a short-term illness, the team of cheerleaders rallies and meets all your needs. Some people love a crisis, so even people who you don't know well will jump in to help. But when there's a recurrence of cancer or when the journey becomes lengthy and discouraging, the friends who thrive in a crisis tend to get tired. As your friend watches this happen, she needs to know that you aren't one of those people who will grow weary of her struggles and move on.

When it becomes clear that there's no chance of a medical cure, some close friends will withdraw in their sadness or fear. A friend of mine who is fighting a second recurrence of cancer told me that some of her long-time friends have "gone silent." It's incredibly painful. She knows that they're scared and don't know how to handle it. They don't know how to walk through this with her, but she needs them now more than ever. She told me, "I wish they would text me and say, 'I'm scared for you.' I wish they would tell me they don't know how to navigate this fear, because I don't know how either."

Your friend may not have the physical or emotional energy to reach out to others, but she'd still like to be included socially. Keep inviting her or initiating time together, even if she has to turn you down. If she feels well while receiving chemo, that could be a great time to visit her. It's no fun getting chemo by yourself, and your presence could give her caregivers a break. Just be sure to bring a book or a magazine and let her know that you'll stay by her side if she needs to take a nap.

Above all, please don't flippantly say that you're praying for her unless it's true. I heard this from many cancer-fighters and caregivers. They are desperate for your prayers and don't want to hear hollow promises. You might even text her and share a Scripture that you've prayed for her. Remember, she needs to know that she's not being forgotten.

Hospice Visits

Typically, when cancer patients decide to discontinue medical treatment to fight the cancer, they enter the care of hospice at home, in a hospital, or at a hospice facility. This is a difficult time for the patient, friends, and family, but it can still be a time of beautiful connection and relationships. I'm going to be blunt: when your friend is in hospice care, she has entered a different phase of her journey, but she is not dead yet. You may feel sad and scared, but please continue showing up for her and her family.

When Jamie's husband was in hospice care, he wanted to spend time with people. Sadly, many people didn't feel comfortable visiting him there, and he knew it. He felt loved when friends came by to visit and acted as upbeat and normal as possible. He didn't need emotional goodbyes. He needed to feel like his friends were just stopping by to say hello, to read something meaningful to him, or to pray with him. It's wise to limit hospice visits to about fifteen minutes, unless you're specifically there to relieve a caregiver. If you're confident that you're in the inner circle of friends, a longer visit may be appropriate. If you aren't sure, at the fifteen-minute mark, offer to leave and let your friend rest, and see if your offer is met with "Thanks for coming" or "Please don't go yet."

When the time comes that your friend receives her heavenly healing and you lose her on earth, please continue to support her family. This will be hard, because you will be grieving, and her family will constantly remind you of your loss. I know that you love your friend, and you can continue to love her beyond her days on earth by serving her family. Your continued presence will communicate volumes to her loved ones and family, reminding them that you love them, too.

When Jean passed away, my routine was left with a gaping hole. My heart hurt. I didn't want to go to her funeral. I wanted to pick up lunch from Panera, drive out to her house on the lake, and chat with my friend.

In a way, my grief felt selfish. For months, I tried to make our visits less about me and more about what she needed. After she died, I focused on my own sadness. But she doesn't need me anymore. She doesn't need anything. She is complete in her Savior. The tears have been wiped from her eyes, and now it's my turn to weep.

And, as I do, I will cling to my Savior, who knows how it feels to weep at the grave of a friend. He knows the pain of death, because he endured it to bring me eternal life. He sees my tears and promises that this hurt won't hurt forever, that this separation is only temporary. Christ alone is the anchor of hope for my grieving heart.

Questions for Reflection

1. What are some ways you can show support to your friend while minimizing her need to respond?
2. What is your friend's mood in her current situation? What tone do you need to match in your communication with her?
3. What are some of your friend's logistical challenges? What are some ways you can help or rally others to help meet her needs?
4. What are your feelings about your friend's prognosis? Who can you trust to listen well and help you process these feelings?

ACTION STEPS TO CONSIDER

☐ Make sure that she knows she is not forgotten, even if her journey becomes long and discouraging.

☐ Regularly communicate support in ways that minimize her need to respond, such as a card in the mail or a meal left on her front porch.

☐ Match her tone: be positive when she's feeling hopeful, acknowledge the reality of her prognosis when she needs to feel understood, and fight alongside her when she's feeling determined.

☐ Regularly offer logistical help. Create a predictable schedule for her helpers so that she knows her needs will be covered and friends won't be overwhelmed.

☐ Continue reaching out, even as the end draws near. Don't let your fear or sadness keep you from initiating time with her, even if she has to turn you down sometimes.

☐ Don't be afraid to visit your friend in hospice care. But keep those visits short unless you are an inner-circle friend or are relieving a caregiver.

☐ I recommend reading the book *Just Show Up*, by Jill Lynn Buteyn and Kara Tippetts, for a further discussion of community and incurable cancer. Resource 3.1 of this book will also help to provide a biblical framework as you suffer alongside your friend.

When It's Not Really Over

Supporting a Friend through Survivorship

In 2011, I wrote this update on my Caring Bridge page:

O magnify the LORD with me,
    and let us exalt his name together! (Ps. 34:3)

I don't know how to write this post without weeping. Which could be kind of embarrassing, since I'm sitting in a Houston-area Panera.

My scan showed that I am CANCER-FREE! Thank you, Lord!

It's a bizarre, happy, wonderful feeling. I can say, "I had cancer." It's past tense. Recurrence will always be a possibility for me (I will return to Houston for scans every three months), but I refuse to live in anxiety about the future. I will only live in today, and today, the cancer is gone. Amazing.

Dr. Ravi has a new nurse since the last time I saw him. The nurse walked us back to the room and said, "I see you have a history of right breast angiosarcoma." It was so strange, because I had never heard anyone say it that way! I like it!

The other news from the appointment is that my platelets are still an issue. Of course! Silly platelets! After hitting 100,000 after surgery (normal is 174,000), they dropped to

70,000 last week and were 57,000 yesterday. Dr. Ravi wants me to follow this closely with my doctor back home and call him if they drop below 40,000. Let's pray they turn around soon!

Because my bone marrow still hasn't recovered from the chemo I finished five months ago, Dr. Ravi has decided not to do any additional chemo. He would have liked to have given me a few more rounds of chemo, but he said it was not necessary and admitted that he's the most aggressive angiosarcoma doctor in the country. I expressed concern that it might not be good that I'm not getting this additional chemo. And his answer was right on: we've done everything we can, and we did a lot, and now we leave it in God's hands. There's no better place to leave it!

So I'm cancer-free, and I don't need any more treatment. I still can't believe it. May God receive all the glory for bringing me through the last ten months. I'm thankful for each and every one of you who have prayed for me, read my journal entries, and served our family. I would appreciate your continued prayers for my bone marrow to recover and that I would never have a recurrence. I'll keep you posted!

I wrote these words at the beginning of my survivorship phase, and they portray the spectrum of emotions that survivors feel as the treatment phase comes to a close. You can tell by my extravagant use of exclamation marks that I was thrilled to be finished with treatment. I was thankful and ecstatic that cancer was now in my past. But you also see that I faced medical challenges with my platelets. I would return for scans every three months in order to check for recurrence. I was concerned about not getting the additional chemo my oncologist had planned. And I was desperate for continued prayers, because I wasn't convinced that cancer would stay in my past.

As I speak to cancer survivors and caregivers, every single one of them affirms this truth: cancer doesn't end when treatment ends. In fact, many survivors will tell you that the first year after cancer treatment is even more difficult than the time they spent fighting cancer. This might surprise you, knowing all that your friend endured during treatment! But survivorship adds new emotional struggles to her lingering physical recovery.

During treatment, we're often in survival mode. We're consumed with attending appointments, managing side effects, watching our blood counts and tumor markers, and trying to meet the basic needs of ourselves and our families. We hate fighting cancer, but we also appreciate fighting the cancer. The fight gives us focus, and we're busy, busy, busy doing something to bring about cancer's demise.

And then it all stops. A doctor tells us we are free to move on with our lives. Or we ring a bell in the chemo room and everyone cheers. Maybe it ends with a surgeon removing the final traces of cancer or repairing the last of the damage it inflicted. Our friends view it as closure and move on to the next crisis, while we're left to cope with the physical, emotional, relational, financial, and spiritual fallout of all we have just experienced. We're expected to return to our pre-cancer life, but nothing feels the same.

Your friend still needs you. Cancer is more than a medical crisis—it's a life-altering, perspective-shifting, relationship-changing experience. Your friend needs your continued support as she navigates the physical, emotional, and relational changes that cancer brought to her life. In this chapter, I hope to help you see what is next for your friend—and how you can continue to love and serve her well.

Your Friend's Changed Body

Many cancer survivors feel that their bodies never return to normal after cancer. We struggle with fatigue, and our blood cell counts (white blood cells, red blood cells, and platelets) may fluctuate for months or even years. We feel foggy and struggle with memory loss due to chemobrain. We miss our pre-cancer hair and struggle to find a short hairstyle that feels right. We have follow-up surgery after breast reconstruction. We endure procedures, surgeries, and various adjustments to the damage that cancer and its treatment left behind.

There is also uncertainty surrounding how to move forward when you aren't seeing a doctor every week. We struggle to walk the fine line between being vigilant about lumps, bumps, aches, and pains that need to be checked out by an oncologist, and all-consuming paranoia. Every headache could be brain cancer. Every backache could be bone metastases. We know we'll sound crazy if we say this aloud. But after the worst-case scenario has played out at least once, your mind is prone to jump to that place every time.

In the year following my treatment, I struggled with the physical changes to my body. At first I was simply thankful to be alive and healthy—I didn't care that I had no hair and one breast. But as time went on, I became discontented with those losses. I longed to wear a cute swimsuit and put my hair in a ponytail. I continued to grieve those physical repercussions.

As I mentioned in chapter 6, I decided to have reconstruction a few years after my mastectomy. I needed three surgeries over the course of seven months, and the appointments and recovery time surrounding these operations consumed much of my time. It was not only a physical challenge but an emotional challenge as well. When friends brought meals, it was a wonderful gift, but it also brought back painful memories. Being dependent on others to care for my kids, feeling tired, sitting in doctors' offices and hospitals—these experiences triggered difficult emotions, despite my enthusiasm for the end result.

In addition to my changed body and short hair, chemo-brain continues to affect my daily life, and I hear this from other survivors as well. Two years after chemo, I was getting my kids settled in our pew, when from the row behind us a friend's husband asked, "Did you and my wife have fun the other night?" I stared at him, completely baffled at the question. What had I done with his wife recently? I had no idea. I thought about just saying that, yes, of course we had fun. But I took the honest approach and asked him to remind me what we had done. The Wednesday before, his wife and I had car-pooled to a church-wide women's meeting. It all came back to me then—and yes, we did have fun! But it was difficult to admit my weakness. I have suffered several embarrassing moments due to my faltering memory and my brain's inability to switch gears quickly. It's frustrating to feel foggy and to lose the sharpness of my pre-cancer mind.

After Samantha's battle with breast cancer in her thirties, she was surprised by how many physical losses she faced. She needed a hysterectomy, and this devastated the plans that she and her husband had to add to their family. They had three children and planned to have another baby close in age to their youngest. It felt as though they lost a child—and it still does. Because she went through menopause early, Samantha feels like an older woman. She wakes up with aches and pains and struggles to style her thinning hair. She can't run like she did before cancer, because radiation damaged her lung. She feels like she missed out on experiencing middle age.

For parents of children with cancer, the long-term phys-ical challenges can be a difficult adjustment. After Pam's young son battled neuroblastoma, her vision for her son's life dramatically changed. Because of his treatment, he wears hearing aids, struggles with athletics, probably cannot have children of his own, and is at risk for other health problems. Pam told me that she tries not to dwell on these problems. She's thankful that her son survived, and she knows it can all change in an instant. But life for her child looks very different than it did before cancer.

These are just a few examples of how life may be different for your friend in ways you can't see. She may or may not talk about these frustrations and losses. But if she does, you'll be prepared not to dismiss her concerns. You'll be ready to listen compassionately, ask questions that express your concern, and offer your support as she navigates these changes.

Your Friend's Changed Emotions

One of the most challenging aspects of cancer survivorship is needing to emotionally process your experience without the same level of support you received when you were fighting cancer. I needed to talk about cancer over and over again. I needed to talk about what I'd been through, how I was still struggling, and my fears for the future. At times I would broach the subject with a friend, and I could see it on her face: *Oh, great—here we go again. More cancer talk. When is she going to move on from this?* Thankfully, I have a wonderful inner circle of friends who compassionately listened to me talk about cancer for years. I also learned to rely more deeply on the Lord, knowing that my friends were finite and would never satisfy my deepest emotional needs.

Cancer survivors also deal with fear about their current and future health. The fear of recurrence sometimes consumes us. It's hard to suddenly be doing nothing medically to prevent the cancer's return. In many cases, the early survivorship months feel less like "I'm cured!" and more like "Let's watch and wait." As your friend watches her community celebrate her health, she may feel cautiously optimistic at best.

It's safest to not assume anything about how your friend feels as her treatment phase ends. Ask questions: How does she feel about finishing treatment? What are her next steps as far as checkups, reconstructive surgery, or maintenance drugs? Is she struggling with physical side effects from treatment? What are her fears or concerns as a cancer survivor? What topics make her want to run screaming from the room? How does it feel to be back to "normal" life?

Medical appointments are never the same again.

Five years after cancer, I was on vacation with my husband when I developed a severe sore throat and had to visit an urgent care clinic. A nurse, who was no doubt grumpy from having to work on a gorgeous Florida Saturday, took me back to get my vitals. She started asking questions.

"Any surgery in the last five years?"

"Well, uh, yes—I had cancer several years ago, and I've had follow-up surgery since then."

I didn't mean to be vague, but my throat felt like it had razor blades sticking through it, and every word hurt. What did my mastectomy in 2011 have to do with my sore throat in 2016?

"What kind of cancer did you have?"

"Angiosarcoma."

Blank stare from the nurse. "So, what kind of surgery did you have?"

"Well . . . several. I had a biopsy, I had a central line inserted, I had a single right mastectomy, and, a few years later, three reconstructive surgeries."

"Oooh," she said condescendingly, "so you had breast cancer."

At this point, I wanted to cry. I wasn't trying to be fancy when I said I had angiosarcoma. It was in my breast (thus the mastectomy), but it wasn't breast cancer, and I won't call it that to a medical professional.

She finally ushered me to an exam room, and a physician's assistant came in. He was intrigued by my chart and wanted to hear all about my angiosarcoma. I didn't feel like sharing my cancer memories with a stranger that day. All I wanted was a strep test and an antibiotic.

When you're a cancer survivor, medical appointments are never the same. Each appointment comes with another medical history form. Check the "cancer" box. List the type and the dates. Regurgitate the well-memorized list of treatments and surgeries with their respective dates. I've experienced serious bouts of anxiety in medical waiting rooms as I fill out those forms and relive the memories.

Medical appointments also stir up fear because it's not a given that I'll walk out of that office without receiving bad news. My doctors are extra-vigilant with me, which I appreciate, but it means that I often experience follow-up tests, blood draws, and biopsies that my doctors wouldn't do for someone who didn't boast a medical history of angiosarcoma. I try to stay optimistic, but those tests can often feel stressful.

There's no anxiety like scanxiety.

When your friend faces a medical appointment for the purpose of monitoring for cancer recurrence, she may feel that she's facing a firing squad. These appointments are so unnerving that the feeling they produce has its own word: Scanxiety. Noun. The unbearable, all-consuming feeling of fear and dread associated with having scans to check for cancer and waiting to receive the results.

Medically, I had a high risk of recurrence in the first few

years. In the beginning, I returned to Houston every three months to be checked for cancer. These visits produced severe anxiety—a medical assistant always took my vitals before I saw the oncologist, and my heart rate was sky high. As soon as I got through each appointment, the next one seemed right around the corner. With a couple of scares from those scans and other symptoms thrown in, I was riding a terrifying emotional roller coaster. My friends learned that even though I was physically healthy, I still needed their emotional support through these ups and downs.

I also struggled to plan anything in the future beyond my next cancer checkup—even details as minor as making lunch plans after a trip to Houston. I felt paralyzed by the uncertainty of what those appointments could bring. When others mentioned an event happening months or even years away, it was painful. Would I be around to enjoy it? How could they live with such confidence? It felt strange that other people thought that way and I didn't. As a cancer survivor, I hesitated to make long-range plans.

Your friend will need your support as she walks through her follow-up surveillance. Doctors turn some survivors loose and say, "Call me if you need anything." Others are monitored closely. Ask if your friend will have medical follow-up appointments. How often will these checkups occur? What tests will she have done? How will she receive the results? How are these appointments affecting her emotionally?

Give lots of grace and space if she struggles emotionally before the appointments. Pam, whose son battled cancer a few years ago, put it this way: "I often feel like a wounded animal, snapping at anyone who comes near me around scan time." I tended to withdraw into my anxiety and dread during the days leading up to my trips to Houston for scans. When your friend's appointments draw near, let her know that you're thinking of her and praying for a good result.

Special occasions bring both joy and sadness.

In the first year following my treatment, I spent each holiday wondering whether I would live to see another one. I put away holiday decorations and prayed I would be the one to get them out the next year. I would wonder what holidays would look like for my family if I wasn't there. Would my husband make sure that the kids had time with my parents and siblings and their families? Would he remember to buy stocking stuffers and teacher gifts? What would happen to our family holiday traditions? I didn't want to waste the holidays feeling sad, but I had to face these fears and emotions in those early years of survivorship.

The one-year anniversary of my diagnosis hit harder than I expected. I felt inundated with memories from the year before—most of which were frightening and sad. The anniversary has gotten easier as time has passed, but those memories are still most potent around that time of year. I was diagnosed on the day of fall parent-teacher conferences at my children's school. Each fall, as the leaves change color and the weather turns cooler, I'm reminded of 2010. My friend Lynette and I still associate parent-teacher conferences with my diagnosis. Every year, we celebrate when I show up to conferences and remember the year I was weeping in my bedroom while she folded my laundry.

I still cry each year on my kids' birthdays. My children assume it's because I don't want them to grow up and leave home, but the truth is that I'm thankful to have survived another year of their lives. Some days, I want time to hurry up so that my children can live as much of their lives as possible with me here. I grateful for each day with my children, but when I watch them blow out the candles each year, it's hard not to think about how greedy I am for more years, more time, more birthdays.

Be aware of the mixed feelings that accompany your friend's holidays, birthdays, and anniversaries. Don't assume that she feels purely celebratory, but don't assume that she's distressed, either. It is likely a mixture of both. Ask questions and let her explain how she feels and how you can support her. Be patient if your friend struggles with mixed emotions surrounding these dates. You may feel that by the second or third anniversary, she should be fine. But remember, this is only the second or third time she has walked through the emotions associated with this particular day. It will get easier, but it will take time.

The future feels impossible.

Your friend may not feel this way, depending on her chances of recurrence and her prognosis. But, for most cancer survivors, the future feels uncertain. I felt like I was standing on a beach in the dark. I could hear the waves rolling in, but I couldn't tell how far out they were or how long it would take for them to come crashing down. Did I have a few healthy months before a recurrence? A year? Could I dare to dream that I might have several healthy years? The uncertainty felt oppressive most days. I found it difficult to act normally around others who didn't feel the same darkness surrounding their future. It's hard to be thirty-five years old and doubt that you'll live to see forty. You're grappling with issues that most of your peers are not.

The year after my cancer battle, my friend's daughter asked me, "Mrs. Marissa, how old will you be when Christopher graduates from high school?" The question shocked me. My first reaction was, *Why would she ask me that? Doesn't she realize I'm not going to live that long?* But, of course, she was only eight years old. She had no idea that her curiosity triggered those emotions. So I did the mental math and answered her question. I would be forty-five years old. And it didn't seem that old. Surely I'd be able to hold on that long, even if the cancer recurred. But at age thirty-five, with a history of angiosarcoma, it felt like too much to hope for. I might as well be trying to live to be a hundred.

My husband has tried to get me to talk about retirement, but I still can't do it. I'm supportive of his financial goals, but I can't discuss our retirement lifestyle. Retirement is way too far into the dark fog of my future. With every healthy year that passes, the fog recedes a little. I start to dream of graduations, weddings, and grandbabies. But the fog is still there, clouding everything.

Remember that your friend is still grieving losses, and her emotional struggles are ongoing. Your friend would likely benefit from professional counseling as she works through these issues. I finally found a counselor one year after I finished treatment—and I wish I had done so much earlier. I needed a place to say things that I couldn't say to my friends for fear of upsetting them. I needed someone to guide me through the grief process. I needed a professional with a biblical view of suffering and God's sovereignty, and I'm thankful that God provided the right person. You may consider suggesting counseling to your friend if you're in her inner circle. (You can even show her this paragraph!) But make sure she knows that you're not trying to pass her off to someone else and that she has your continued emotional support.

Your Friend's Changed Friendships

Because of the intense nature of my treatment and the large amount of time I spent in Houston, I felt like I was reentering my social world after being in a cave for nine months. My friends had changed, and some of the relationships among my circle of friends had changed. Because I hadn't been there to see it happen gradually, it seemed foreign and sudden. I was accustomed to being alone and focusing on my survival, so it took time for me to adjust to being in two-way relationships again. It took awhile for me to stop being self-absorbed and to maintain balanced friendships, especially when I was still feeling so emotionally needy.

The fears and emotions that I struggled with in my early years of survivorship sometimes caused me to feel isolated in my friendships. I remember one girls' night out in the first year or two after cancer. Although my oldest wasn't yet a tween, some of my friends had older kids, and the conversation turned to topics related to raising teens. I wanted to run screaming from the table, because I didn't think I would live to parent a teenager. I wondered who would talk to my sons about how to treat girls or take my daughter to buy her first bra. I couldn't handle the cavalier way that my friends talked about the future. It made me feel different, jealous, and sad.

I didn't want friends to feel nervous around me or to constantly fear they would say something to trigger hard emotions. So I hid my struggles from those outside my inner circle. But I needed my close friends to understand the truth. I needed them to catch my eye in a group of acquaintances when the chatter turned to having "the talk" with our kids, our aging bodies, or next summer's vacation plans. I needed them to reach out with support when I wanted to withdraw before each Houston checkup. I needed to know that they hadn't moved on—that they were still with me for the long haul.

In addition to my close friends, I felt safest with other cancer survivors. They knew not to talk too far in the future. They related to the fear and sadness I felt. They were understanding and safe. We had an instant bond that led to close friendships. But being friends with cancer survivors isn't easy. Some of my friends have endured recurrences. It's devastating to watch someone who you care about walk through your worst nightmare. I've been active at times in a Facebook group for angiosarcoma patients, survivors, and caregivers. I love the relationships and the sense of camaraderie. But, if I'm honest, there are seasons when it's too difficult for me to handle the bad news and losses in the group.

Your friend may or may not choose to seek support among other cancer survivors. Don't force her into it. But if she suddenly has a new group of friends, don't feel threatened. I would have understood if my new friendships had bothered my close friends who put their lives on hold to serve me. But if it did, they never let on. They were supportive of those new friendships and the comfort that they brought me.

As the friend of a cancer survivor, you can take tangible steps to celebrate your friend's survivorship. You could participate in cancer-research fundraisers in her honor or acknowledge the awareness month for her type of cancer. Or put her diagnosis anniversary on your calendar each year and send her flowers or a card to mark another year of survivorship.

Your Friend's Changed Perspective

Yes, the challenges of cancer survivorship are many. But so are the blessings. Sometimes I wonder: what if the biopsy result had gone the other way? What if the phone call had confirmed that the lump in my breast was a simple infection? What if I'd never experienced cancer? I'm thankful that God didn't let me choose the outcome of my biopsy in October 2010. I would have chosen the easier road of a benign result. I would have missed all that he's been faithful to teach me and the ways that he's used my suffering for good. I'd have missed the new perspective that cancer brings.

It feels like my future is covered in darkness, and that is hard. But there's a sense in which I see a reality that many women my age do not: our time on this earth is finite and uncertain. This understanding drives me to be more intentional in my marriage, parenting, and other relationships. In the early months and years of survivorship, I focused on making memories with my family and pouring into their lives as much as possible. I was racing against a stopwatch with an unknown amount of time. Thankfully, my experience with cancer zeroed my focus onto the truth of God's character. I knew that, no matter what my kids faced in the future, they needed to understand who God says he is and what he promises in his Word. I was relentless in teaching my children these truths.

I was also an obnoxiously fun mom. (My kid's friends often complained that their moms weren't nearly as fun.) I created so many new family traditions that I could hardly keep track of them all! We laughed, played, and ate a lot of ice cream. I was obsessed with making up for lost time and for future time that I was afraid we might not have. But I'll never regret the time I spent focused on enjoying life with my kids while they were young. I knew not to wish those months and years away, waiting for things to get easier. Yes, we had tough days. It wasn't all sunshine and rainbows and sundaes every day. But I was thankful, and I knew that each day was precious.

Cancer also brings a new spiritual perspective. I know what it feels like to have been prayed for by people I've never met. I know the sweet closeness of the Lord in the midst of a trial. I know the assurance of salvation that comes from seeing the Spirit at work in my life and knowing without a doubt that he lives in me. I'll share more of these benefits of suffering in Resource 3.1, and I hope you will take the time to read it and be encouraged. We'll discuss how God hates suffering, but how he also brings good into our lives even in our heartbreak. I know, because I lived it.

I look at my past and know that his faithfulness is real. I look at my present and know that his faithfulness is true. And I look at the cross and know that his faithfulness exceeds my human understanding. So I can face an uncertain future, knowing that I belong to a faithful Father who loves me.

Questions for Reflection

1. Which aspects of the description of survivorship do you think apply to your friend's situation?
2. How has your friend expressed difficulty in navigating survivorship?
3. Which specific ways to support a survivor stood out to you? How can you put these ideas into action?

ACTION STEPS TO CONSIDER

☐ Ask your friend how she feels about her treatment coming to an end. Find out what physical side effects or changes she's adjusting to, what her fears are, and how you can continue to provide support.

☐ Remember her ongoing losses and grief process. Let her know you are in it for the long haul and are aware of her struggles.

☐ Know her schedule for medical follow-up appointments and what they involve.

☐ Encourage her continued emotional healing, which may include professional counseling and connecting with other survivors.

☐ Be aware of the mixed feelings she may experience around holidays, birthdays, and anniversaries.

☐ Celebrate her survivorship by participating in research fundraisers in her honor, marking her survivorship anniversary, or acknowledging the awareness month for her type of cancer.

Practical Support Resources

Forms and Readings for Helping Your Friend

Resource 1.1

Resources to Help Your Friend

As you start thinking about ways to help your friend, use this sheet to brainstorm resources that are available to you. This can include other friends!

Tangible	Emotional	Spiritual

Resource 2.1

A Biblical View of Community

In this resource and Resource 3.1, we will discuss community and suffering in light of God's Word. This is the theological foundation for the practical applications we've discussed in this book. These resources aren't meant to be exhaustive discussions of these topics. They aren't a deep dive into complicated issues and questions; they're more like a snorkeling expedition on which we'll gaze at relevant truths from Scripture and be encouraged to serve our friends with these truths in mind.

The Mandate and Privilege of Christian Community

"I know why that big house of yours is called a sorority. It's a house of sisters."

This is how my middle child greeted his favorite babysitter one day. After attending "Chicken Finger Friday" at her sorority house, he was intensely curious about this large house of girls. But it's tough to explain a sorority to a five-year-old boy. Then, at school, they learned the Latin words for family members. Sister in Latin is *soror*. All of a sudden, it clicked: a house of sisters.

In a college sorority, a group of young women live together, united by their pledge to the sorority. They may have common interests, but they also have different majors, backgrounds, skills, struggles, opinions, and expectations. Because each one is in the sorority, they are bound together. They are sisters.

Paul teaches us in 1 Corinthians that the same is true of

us as Christians. Just as a young woman can't be in a sorority without others, we aren't Christians on our own. There's no such thing as a lone Christian. If you are in Christ, you are in Christ with others. We are bound together by our belonging to him. We aren't part of the body of Christ just at certain times or in certain seasons—we are always part of the body of Christ, even when it's tough.

First Corinthians 12:12–13 says:

> For just as the body is one and has many members, and all the members of the body, though many, are one body, so it is with Christ. For in one Spirit we were all baptized into one body—Jews or Greeks, slaves or free—and all were made to drink of one Spirit.

The Spirit that dwells in me also dwells in you. And in a believer on the other side of the world. And in believers throughout other times in history—past, present, and future. This Spirit unites all believers into one invisible church, which is the body of Christ. Though there are many members, and though we have differences, we are all one body.

If the Holy Spirit dwells in you—if you are in Christ—then this truth is your reality: you are not doing the Christian life on your own. You are a Christian in a spiritual community.

Christian community isn't just a mandate; it's a gift. If you live in a country where Christians are free to meet together, you have the privilege of physical Christian community. In Dietrich Bonhoeffer's classic work *Life Together*, he writes about this gift: "So between the death of Christ and the Last Day it is only by a gracious anticipation of the last things that Christians are privileged to live in visible fellowship with other Christians. It is by the grace of God that a congregation is permitted to gather visibly in this world to share God's Word and sacrament."[1] When Christ returns, the invisible church will be able to assemble together—every last one of us. In the meantime, we're scattered around the globe. Many believers do not freely enjoy fellowship like American Christians do, so any time that we spend together physically—"visibly," as Bonhoeffer said—is precious and powerful. As we will see throughout this resource, God pours out gifts to his children through the body of Christ. As we worship, hear the Word preached, partake of the Lord's Supper, and fellowship together, God uses time with our brothers and sisters in Christ to strengthen our faith.

If we avoid community, we forsake the body of Christ. We miss out on the gifts that he gives us through that community. A biblical Christian life is lived in community with others.

The Characteristics of Christian Community

Christian community is complex, and we won't explore all its facets in this resource. This brief flyover of foundational truth will inform our actions as we seek to serve our friends who have cancer. I'd like to draw your attention to four key characteristics of Christian community. From Scripture we see that, as a Christian community, we love lavishly, serve sacrificially, grow in the gospel, and embrace each other's emotions.

In Christian community, we love lavishly.

In John 13, Jesus tells his disciples, "A new commandment I give to you, that you love one another: just as I have loved you, you also are to love one another. By this all people will know that you are my disciples, if you have love for one another" (vv. 34–35). When we love our brothers and sisters in Christ, we are fulfilling Christ's command. But we aren't simply to love them; we are commanded to love as Christ loved us.

How did Christ love us? He humbled himself to dwell

among us so he could sympathize with our weakness (see Heb. 4:15). He traded the glory of heaven for a life spent serving others, washing the feet of his betrayer, and giving his life for us (see John 13; Phil. 2:5–8). When we were his enemies, he suffered and died for us (see Rom. 5:8). He "came not to be served but to serve, and to give his life as a ransom for many" (Mark 10:45). This is the lavish love with which Christ loves us. This is the lavish love with which we are to love our brothers and sisters in Christ. This is the lavish love that characterizes Christian community.

In Christian community, we serve sacrificially.

In John 13, Jesus gives us an example of how to serve others. As the disciples gathered for the Passover meal, there was one job no one wanted. I imagine they started looking around at each other, each one considering his position in the group. Who was the lowest guy on the totem pole? Who would end up with the job of washing the filthy feet of his friends? They never imagined that Jesus would be the one to grab the rags and the bowl of water. They couldn't believe their eyes as he knelt in front of them, one by one, and washed the mess from their feet.

> When he had washed their feet and put on his outer garments and resumed his place, he said to them, "Do you understand what I have done to you? You call me Teacher and Lord, and you are right, for so I am. If I then, your Lord and Teacher, have washed your feet, you also ought to wash one another's feet. For I have given you an example, that you also should do just as I have done to you. Truly, truly, I say to you, a servant is not greater than his master, nor is a messenger greater than the one who sent him. If you know these things, blessed are you if you do them." (vv. 12–17)

Jesus didn't wash the disciples' feet for the sake of a poignant moment or surprising anecdote. He washed their feet in order to give them an example. He wanted them to understand that no act of service was below them. Every task, no matter how humiliating, could be yours if you're a follower of Christ. We are called to serve our brothers and sisters sacrificially.

In Christian community, we grow in the gospel.

Part of living in Christian community is bringing each other to Jesus. Just as the friends of the paralytic in Mark 2 went to great lengths to bring their friend to Jesus, we must also bring our friends to the living Word of God. We know some who are further along in their understanding of God's Word, and they can help us move forward. We meet others who are less mature, and we can spur them on. We need one another. We all have a role to play in helping one another grow.

Hebrews 10:24–25 says, "And let us consider how to stir up one another to love and good works, not neglecting to meet together, as is the habit of some, but encouraging one another, and all the more as you see the Day drawing near." Part of living in Christian community is spurring one another on in the Christian life. I have days when I need encouragement. I have days when I'm the encourager. Every day, I need others, and they need me. Jesus didn't intend for us to do this alone. He didn't intend for us to struggle with sin on our own or seek to understand the gospel without someone to guide, instruct, and counsel us. He gave us the body of Christ so that we could help one another grow into the likeness of Christ.

In Christian community, we embrace each other's emotions.

If one part of your body hurts, you hurt. When you have strep throat, you don't say, "Well, my throat is sick. But the rest of me is just fine." No! You say, "I'm sick! Pass the antibiotics, please!" Likewise, if one member of the body of Christ hurts, the entire body feels that pain. First Corinthians 12:26 tells us, "If one member suffers, all suffer together; if one member is honored, all rejoice together." Hebrews 13:3 says, "Remember those who are in prison, as though in prison with them, and those who are mistreated, since you also are in the body." When a brother is in prison, it is as if we are in prison with him. This is what it means to be the body of Christ.

One way that we live out Christian community with those who are hurting is to embrace their emotions with empathy and comfort. We don't deny their pain; we share it. Romans 12:15 tells us to "rejoice with those who rejoice, weep with those who weep." If we are going to weep with those who suffer, we must first acknowledge their pain. The body of Christ should be a place where empathy abounds. In *The Listening Life*, Adam McHugh says, "The church is a community of people who acknowledge suffering, treat it as real and enter into one another's pain, because our Lord knows our afflictions. Jesus offers his presence in suffering, and so should we."[2]

We share in one another's suffering, and we also share in one another's comfort. When God comforts me, he doesn't intend that comfort just for me. God comforts me so that I can comfort others in the body. As I embrace my sisters' emotions, I have a gift of comfort to share with them from my own experience of comfort. When your mouth swallows an antibiotic, it enters your bloodstream, and your blood carries it to the body part that hurts. Similarly, God gives comfort to one member of the body who carries it to another member who is hurting. To do our job properly, we must enter into the suffering of others in order to carry comfort to them.

Second Corinthians 1:3–4 says,

> Blessed be the God and Father of our Lord Jesus Christ, the
> Father of mercies and God of all comfort, who comforts us
> in all our affliction, so that we may be able to comfort those
> who are in any affliction, with the comfort with which we
> ourselves are comforted by God.

Tim Keller describes church as "a community of profound
consolation."[3] What if the church was the first place that hurting people went to for comfort? What if our neighbors saw
the church as a place of refuge for suffering people to rest in
the empathetic, comforting arms of the body of Christ? God's
Word calls us to be that type of community.

When I battled cancer, my community loved me lavishly,
served me sacrificially, helped me to grow in the gospel, and
embraced my emotions. I needed to have reasonable expectations of those around me and put my trust in the Lord, not my
friends, to meet my needs. But, over and over again, I saw God
provide for me through the body of Christ. Christian community served a vital role in God's plan for my cancer journey.

The Obstacles to Christian Community

When I started writing about how my friends supported
me through cancer, most of the response I received was positive and encouraging. Many women with cancer are being
loved well by their church families. But I received one response
that devastated me. A cancer-fighting friend wrote to tell me
that she had to stop reading my story. She was not receiving
the same level of support that I received, and hearing my experience made her feel angry and resentful.

Her feedback made me wonder: what's causing the dis-
connect between the church's desire to care for the sick and
the experience of one who doesn't feel cared for? Maybe you

wondered this, too, as you read the characteristics of Christian community that I just described. Maybe you thought of ways your community is lacking or has disappointed you in the past. Maybe you even had a sinking feeling that you've let your community down sometimes.

There isn't a simple answer to this problem—these situations are multifaceted. But I see two primary obstacles standing in the way of biblical community. I hope that, by bringing these to your attention, I'll encourage you to examine yourself and move past these obstacles in your life, for the benefit of your local church. These two obstacles are busyness and fear.

Community is inconvenient and time-consuming. And we are so, *so* busy. God's Word exhorts us to be busy with knowing and serving and encouraging others. But we're consumed by the demands of other priorities. How can you take a meal to a sister in Christ if you're shuttling kids to practice every afternoon? How can you take time to listen to a friend's struggle when there's not an hour of spare time in your week to meet for coffee? How can you build intentional relationships with a small group of believers when you're constantly chasing other pursuits? We structure our time according to our priorities, and, too often, Christian community doesn't rank high on the list. We need to take an honest look at what our calendars reveal about our priorities and ask the Lord for guidance.

Living in community with others is also risky, and risk is frightening. We're afraid of being known by others. We don't want them to see the mess inside our hearts and our families. We're also afraid of knowing others and their messes. Life in Christian community might require us to hear some things that make us squirm. We might be drawn into the struggles of other people—which could make us uncomfortable or inconvenienced. It's much easier and safer to maintain our carefully crafted facades and not unwrap the junk that hides inside. Our fear drives us to keep all interactions at a superficial level, but Christian community doesn't happen there.

As Christians, we need our community, and our community needs us. If we neglect community because of busyness or fear, there are negative consequences for us, for the community, and for those who desperately need our care. As we address these issues in our hearts and lives, I hope we will all benefit from the stronger communities that result.

The Gift of Christian Community

Although no church is perfect, many imperfect Christian communities heed the call to minister to those in their midst. The church continues to be a place where the poor, sick, and needy are cared for—whether their needs are spiritual, physical, or emotional. When we engage in community with other believers, we experience the gifts of Christian community. Many of the blessings that God gives can come to us only through the body of Christ. These gifts are many, and I'll highlight a few of them here.

Christian community reminds us of our need for grace and truth.

There are some mornings when I think I've got my sin under control. But then I walk out of my bedroom and interact with my family. Most days, it doesn't take long for my sinful tendencies to show. Being in community with others shines a spotlight on my selfishness, impatience, irritability, unkindness, and so much more. I cannot keep Christ's command to love others as myself. I need the Holy Spirit at work in me, producing his fruit in me. I need God's grace and forgiveness. I need Christ's righteousness to cover all my shortcomings.

And so Christian community pushes us deeper into our relationship with the Lord and dependence on him.

Our brothers and sisters in Christ also remind us of our need for biblical truth. One of my closest friends often says to me, "Tell me something true about God." She knows what she needs, but she can't provide it for herself when she's struggling. Yes, the Holy Spirit dwells in her, but sometimes God brings her comfort through other people speaking the truth to her. And my friend isn't ashamed to reach out to believers and ask for comfort.

Bonhoeffer describes it this way: "The Christ in his own heart is weaker than the Christ in the word of his brother; his own heart is uncertain, his brother's is sure."[4] When our heart is uncertain, we need our friends to be sure for us. When our faith is weak, we need others to be strong. It's an important function of Christian community and a gift from the Lord when we provide comfort, hope, and encouragement to our hurting brothers and sisters.

Christian community provides encouragement for our struggles.

In his book *Being There*, Dave Furman writes about his need for encouragement: "I need to be reminded of God's sovereign goodness. And those reminders often come through my friends who turn out to be not just friends but hope dealers."[5] In Christian community, the Lord gives us friends who are hope dealers. Bonhoeffer also exhorts us to speak God's Word to each other. He says that we need to hear the truth from our brothers and sisters over and over again in times of discouragement and doubt.[6]

I recently spent a cold winter morning at a coffee shop with two friends. First I spent an hour with my friend Lynette. She was having a great week, but I was a mess. She listened thoughtfully as I unloaded my troubles on her, gave wise counsel, and cheered my heart. Then our mutual friend Ashley arrived to meet me. The three of us chatted briefly, and I told Ashley how Lynette had encouraged me. I said, "Now I'm ready to encourage you if you're a mess today." Ashley's eyes filled with tears as she replied, "Oh, that's good. Because I'm really a mess."

Ecclesiastes 4:9–10 says,

> Two are better than one, because they have a good reward for their toil. For if they fall, one will lift up his fellow. But woe to him who is alone when he falls and has not another to lift him up!

That morning in the coffee shop, Lynette lifted me up. Then I had a hand to offer Ashley when she was down. We were hope dealers to each other. I desperately needed this gift of Christian community when I battled cancer, and I'm still thankful for my hope dealers today.

Christian community helps us share each other's burdens.

More than once, I've woken up with a sore back because I decided to move a piece of furniture by myself. I'm stubborn when it comes to moving heavy objects. I hate to ask for help, and at first the load never seems too heavy. I'm confident that I can handle it. The next day, my throbbing back tells a different story. But if I ask for help and allow someone to help me, the weight becomes bearable. The load is still heavy, but I know that we'll get the job done without hurting ourselves.

Galatians 6:2 says, "Bear one another's burdens, and so fulfill the law of Christ." Some days we can manage with just a hand to help us. But other days the weight of the mess we're carrying is so heavy, we can't manage it alone. We need our brothers and sisters to come alongside us and take some of the load on themselves.

This means that in Christian community, we never suffer alone. We suffer and struggle together. The young wife who is grieving a miscarriage doesn't grieve alone. The man who is struggling with unemployment doesn't struggle alone. The salvation of a prodigal child doesn't weigh only on the minds of his parents but tops the prayer list of the entire community. Similarly, I didn't battle cancer alone. The tumor was in my body, but the cancer experience was shared throughout the body of Christ. The other members made sacrifices to help me bear my burden.

When we share a brother or sister's burden, Galatians 6:2 says that we "fulfill the law of Christ." This is how we keep Christ's command in John 13:34 to love one another as he loved us. Carrying the burdens of others is not easy. It's often inconvenient. When we're carrying a shoebox and someone else is carrying an elephant, we might need to set our box down—i.e., let some items on our to-do list wait awhile—and serve her sacrificially. Let the dishes sit in your sink while you take groceries to a homebound friend. Skip your weekly latte and buy a gas card for a single mom. When you do, the Lord works through you to give one of his children a lighter burden. Your friend experiences one of the gifts of Christian community, and God is glorified by your obedience.

What about Our Non-Christian Friends?

This book is written primarily for believers with believing friends, and I hope that your friend with cancer shares your faith in Christ. If she doesn't, you have a weighty and wonderful opportunity to put the love of Christ on display before her. Our lavish love and sacrificial service extend beyond the body of Christ to all our neighbors. As John 13:35 reminds us, a watching world sees evidence of our belonging to Christ when we love others. Paul exhorts us to serve others in order to win the lost to Christ in 1 Corinthians 9:19: "For though I am free from all, I have made myself a servant to all, that I might win more of them."

Consider these additional exhortations from Scripture:

Let no one seek his own good, but the good of his neighbor. (1 Cor. 10:24)

Let each of you look not only to his own interests, but also to the interests of others. (Phil. 2:4)

So then, as we have opportunity, let us do good to everyone, and especially to those who are of the household of faith. (Gal. 6:10)

See that no one repays anyone evil for evil, but always seek to do good to one another and to everyone. (1 Thess. 5:15)

And so we have a responsibility first to our Christian community (the household of faith), but then also to those who are apart from Christ. As we love and serve, we can also share the hope that we have in Christ and can pray for our friend's salvation and inclusion in the body of Christ. If your friend is a believer who's been disillusioned by her past experience with the church, pray for her return to Christian fellowship. Encourage her to find a healthy local church where she can experience the gifts of community.

Practically speaking, you'll need to filter some of the advice that is given in this book through your personal knowledge of your friend. There are many suggestions that apply to believing and unbelieving friends, but you may need to thoughtfully tailor your support to your friend's worldview.

I learned from my son that *soror* means sister, and according to the Oxford Latin Dictionary the root word of community is *communitas*, which means "joint possession, partnership; fellowship, kinship."[7] As a Christian community, we share our joys, sorrows, challenges, and victories. And through it all we have fellowship in our Lord and Savior, Jesus Christ, and shared possession of all God's promises in him. Let's recognize the gift of biblical community and our desperate need of it. Let's live out lavish love, sacrificial service, growth in the gospel, and the embracing of one another's emotions. Let's throw aside fear and busyness. Let's enjoy the gifts of sanctification, encouragement, and shared burdens. Let's live out the reality of life together in Christ—a life in which no one suffers alone.

Questions for Reflection

1. What was new or interesting to you about the mandate and privilege of Christian community?
2. Which characteristics of Christian community have you enjoyed in the past? Which have been lacking in your Christian communities?
3. How can you help provide the gifts of community to your suffering friend?

Resource 2.2

A Letter to Your Husband about Her Husband

"Hey, man—how're you doing? Everything good? Okay, great; good to see you!"

My husband stared at the retreating back of the guy who had just slapped him on the back in the church lobby. His friend hurriedly spoke these words and kept walking. My husband wanted to yell after him, "No, everything is not good! My wife has cancer, and I feel like I'm drowning!" But he learned quickly that, even at church, few men took the time to ask meaningful questions and listen to his answers. He watched cards flood our mailbox—mostly ones that were addressed to me. My phone buzzed continuously, but his was mostly silent.

It didn't bother him much—he wasn't sure what he would say even if they asked. And he knew that he wouldn't know what to say if the roles were reversed and Mr. Slap-on-the-Back's wife were in Houston fighting for her life. But as I've spoken with other husbands, I've heard similar stories. Most men are not receiving the support that they need. We need to do a better job of surrounding men with a caring community as they walk this difficult road with their wives.

In this resource, we'll take a look at what cancer feels like to the husbands of cancer-fighters. Feel free to hand the book to your man for a while so that he can learn how to support your friend's husband through her battle. (Seriously. Hand it over now, please!)

Guys, this part is for you. So when I say "your friend," I'm referring to the husband of a cancer patient. Let's chat about what your friend is going through and how you can help. Support looks different for men, but it's still important and necessary.

What He's Experiencing

He's lonely.

When Mike's wife received treatment for breast cancer, he felt like a single parent. His wife spent weeks receiving treatment in another state. When she was home, she was often in bed or facing physical limitations that kept her from her typical lifestyle and responsibilities. He missed her presence. He missed her partnership. Her absence and illness prevented him from seeing friends as often as he had before cancer, compounding his loneliness.

He's in survival mode.

Your friend is probably desperate to love and protect his family, but that requires a great deal of extra effort these days. He's taking on new responsibilities at home, especially if they have young children. He may be worn out by all that needs to be done.

Mike told me that when his wife had cancer, he felt like he was working nonstop, and yet he was spending less time at work and not working as well. He said, "I was exhausted and overwhelmed and yet felt like I was failing at work. I wondered if others resented having to pick up my slack." He needed help, but he was torn between wanting to ask and wanting to be able to handle it all on his own.

He's grieving.

Even when the prognosis is positive, cancer brings a great sense of loss. Your wife and I talked about these losses throughout this book, so I'll let her fill you in. Be aware that your friend is dealing with loss, sadness, and grief, even if his wife is likely to survive her illness. Grieving men may appear sad, scattered, or even rude. Treat him with grace and patience as he processes all that his family is enduring.

What He Needs

He needs your prayers.

Ask your friend how you can pray for him, and then do it. Depending on your relationship, you may decide to pray with him in person. If you pray for him on your own, let him know that you're praying with a text or an email. The ideas I gave your wife in chapter 10 about how to pray for her friend may give you ideas as well.

He needs a break.

Your friend needs time to do something he enjoys so that he can be effective as a caregiver for his spouse and children. This might be time with the Lord, exercise, or an outing with friends. Don't be afraid to take him away from caregiving and spend time with him fishing, hiking, or doing any other activity he enjoys. One husband told me, "You can't underestimate the value in a change of scenery, a listening ear, some good food, and humor."

You may need to help with the logistics of finding a substitute caregiver so that he can get time away. Arrange a babysitter or ask your wife to stay at their house while you take him out for some guy time.

He needs a listening ear.

He may see people avoiding him and feel like a leper. He knows that most guys aren't comfortable talking about cancer.

You can support him by being willing to talk about whatever is on his mind. He doesn't need insightful advice or rehearsed words of comfort. Just be present, acknowledge the situation, and then be available to listen. If he doesn't open up, don't take it personally. He may need a break from the topic today.

He needs friends who care.

Your friend needs to know your concern for him. You can encourage him with a letter or card in the mail. If you don't feel comfortable with words, ask your wife to write a note—but be sure that she addresses it to the cancer-fighter *and* her husband. You should also check on your friend regularly so he doesn't feel forgotten. Keep asking him to go out, even if he says he doesn't need it. Force him to slow down and accept help. But don't get your feelings hurt if he doesn't respond to your offers. Just keep reaching out and letting him know you care.

He needs financial support.

I asked Mike, "What's the best way to offer to help with finances?" He replied, "With a check!" Realize that a cancer battle is typically expensive, and the husband might bear the weight of the financial burden. If you worry that he might be too embarrassed to accept a check in person, consider sending it in the mail. Make sure that he knows it is freely given without any strings attached, and that his family is free to use it for whatever they choose.

Don't forget to look around your community and see whom you can bring along with you to give support. Do you know other men who could pool their money for gift cards? Coworkers who could donate their paid vacation days? Is there a group who could organize a fundraiser or a time of prayer? Remember that you're not alone in supporting your friend. You are one link in his support chain.

Guys, thank you for being willing to risk awkward inter-actions in order to meet your friend's needs. I know that this isn't easy for any of you. Your friend may not say it, but he's thankful for your love and concern.

A Biblical View of Suffering

On the Sunday after my diagnosis, I stood in church next to my husband, singing "In Christ Alone." The words and music washed peace and comfort over my hurting soul. But, at the same time, singing about hope in a storm brought my pain to the surface. Halfway through the song, my husband sat back down in the pew, his face in his hands, as if he couldn't stand any longer under the burden he shouldered.

I remained standing, partly because if I let my tears loose they might never stop, and partly because I wanted to prove my strength. Like many Christians, I equated faith with unwavering, smiling acceptance of hardship. I was uncomfortable with the raw emotions of suffering. I was eager to find the silver lining for myself and others. I believed that nicely packaged suffering would be better received than the mess of grief and fear that I felt. I wanted to encourage others through my suffering, not to bring them down into my pain.

But I was wrong. I underestimated how much others could learn from the Lord in the pit of my pain. As I walked further into my cancer experience, God taught me more about himself and his involvement with our suffering. I learned to stop ignoring my hard emotions and to run to the Lord with them instead. He heals our shattered hearts, but first we need to admit we are broken.

During my illness, I needed God's Word to sustain me. I also craved a deeper understanding of suffering as I wrestled with the turn my life had taken. A friend gave me *A Place of Healing* by Joni Eareckson Tada, and it was one of the few books that brought comfort in my pain. After my medical treatment ended, I wanted to learn more. In this resource, I'll be quoting from two books that have shaped my view of God and suffering: *Walking with God through Pain and Suffering*, by Timothy Keller, and *Be Still, My Soul*, edited by Nancy Guthrie. We will explore the role of God the Father, Son, and Holy Spirit in our suffering, how God uses our suffering, and how we can walk with God in suffering.

The Role of God in Our Suffering

God is not a detached observer of our suffering, watching from above as we try to figure out the trials of life. He does not wring his hands with worry or cross his fingers for us and hope that we'll pull through. He is the Creator and Sustainer of the universe, the sovereign and almighty Lord, and our compassionate heavenly Father. We see in Scripture that all three persons of the Trinity—Father, Son, and Holy Spirit— are intimately involved with our suffering.

God the Father hates suffering.

The Father hates cancer and death. When Adam sinned, evil and suffering entered the good world that God created (see Gen. 3). This was a turning point for humanity. Our relationships with God, creation, and each other were broken. But amidst the curse of pain and death was a promise. The Lord told the serpent that a redeemer would come: "I will put enmity between you and the woman, and between your offspring and her offspring; he shall bruise your head, and you shall bruise his heel" (Gen. 3:15).

God proved his hatred for suffering when he sent his Son to defeat it on the cross. Christ's triumph over evil is a past, present, and future reality. Colossians 2:15 tells us that, on the cross, God "disarmed the rulers and authorities and put them to open shame, by triumphing over them in [Christ]." In this past event, God triumphed over the devil. First Corinthians 15:25–26 says,

> For he must reign until he has put all his enemies under his feet. The last enemy to be destroyed is death.

Jesus is now reigning and working to defeat his enemies. Verse 54 of the same chapter tells us, "When the perishable puts on the imperishable, and the mortal puts on immortality, then shall come to pass the saying that is written: 'Death is swallowed up in victory.'" In the future, when Christ returns, death will be swallowed up in victory and will no longer touch those who are in Christ.

Satan has been defeated. His doom is sure, and Christ's victory is certain (see Rev. 20:1–10; 22:3–7). And yet we live in a fallen world, where God assures us that we will suffer (see John 16:33). Some days it feels like evil is winning. But God reigns over all, and he uses the suffering that he hates to accomplish good in the lives of his people (see Rom. 8:28).

God the Son entered into our suffering.

God the Son not only cares about our suffering but also understands our suffering. When Jesus Christ took on flesh and walked on earth, he suffered. He didn't only suffer on the cross— he suffered loss and betrayal and pain prior to the anguish of Calvary. Isaiah 53:3 prophetically speaks of Jesus when it says that he was "a man of sorrows and acquainted with grief."

Jesus was led by the Spirit into the wilderness, where he fasted for forty days and nights. Matthew 4:2 casually mentions that at the end of this time he was hungry. Jesus was fully divine and also fully human. I expect that, after forty days in the wilderness with no food, saying that he was hungry is quite the understatement! He suffered physically and then suffered spiritually as he faced Satan's temptations in the wilderness.

Jesus also suffered emotional pain. He wept at the tomb of his dear friend, Lazarus. The Son knew the Father's plans and trusted the Father completely. And yet, when Jesus arrived at the tomb of his friend Lazarus and saw the grieving crowd, he didn't chastise them for a lack of faith. He wept with them. He shared in their suffering. Before he encouraged them with the truth that he is the resurrection and the life, he grieved with them (see John 11:17–44).

Jesus wept over Jerusalem, her faithlessness, and her future (see Luke 19:41–44). He was betrayed by one of his twelve closest friends—one of the companions who had walked beside him for three years of public ministry (see Matt. 26:47–50). Jesus wept in the garden of Gethsemane before going to the cross. He submitted to the Father's will, but he didn't go to the cross skipping and whistling. His suffering was real. He wrestled with the hardship he faced. He placed his life in the hands of his Father, but his trust was accompanied by tears (see Matt. 26:36–46).

On the cross, Jesus experienced physical, emotional, and spiritual suffering. The whip hitting his back, the thorns piercing his brow, the nails in his hands, his ribs straining under the pressure, slow suffocation to the point of death—we will never experience the physical suffering that he took for us. He looked down from the cross to see that most of his friends and followers had abandoned him. He was mocked by those next to him and those who were crucifying him. And the greatest suffering of all came when the Father turned his back on the Son, and Jesus cried out, "My God, my God, why have you forsaken me?" (see Matt. 27; Mark 15; Luke 23; John 19). Our Savior suffered in order to spare us the pain of separation from God and to demonstrate his love for us.

In Tim Keller's book on suffering, he writes that we don't know why there is suffering in the world, but we know that it's not because God doesn't love us. He says, "It cannot be that he does not care. He is so committed to our ultimate happiness that he was willing to plunge into the greatest depths of suffering himself."[1] This truth brings comfort when we encounter trials. When we are tempted to question God's love for us, we can look to the cross and know the depth of his steadfast love.

This truth also draws us to our Savior's throne of grace in our suffering. Because he was forsaken by God the Father, we never will be (see Matt 27:46; Heb. 13:5). We are invited to bring our troubles to him with confidence in his grace and mercy:

> For we do not have a high priest who is unable to sympathize with our weaknesses, but one who in every respect has been tempted as we are, yet without sin. Let us then with confidence draw near to the throne of grace, that we may receive mercy and find grace to help in time of need. (Heb. 4:15–16)

God the Spirit comforts us in our suffering.

The Holy Spirit has been given to us by the Father to remind us of the truth of God's Word and his promises. In John 14:26, Jesus tells his disciples, "But the Helper, the Holy Spirit, whom the Father will send in my name, he will teach you all things and bring to your remembrance all that I have said to you." The Spirit plants God's Word deep in the soil of our hearts and minds so that, when trials come, we are rooted in the truth. He does this in several ways.

First, the Spirit pours God's love into our hearts. Romans 5:5 teaches us that the Holy Spirit brings us steadfast hope in the midst of suffering, "and hope does not put us to shame, because God's love has been poured into our hearts through the Holy Spirit who has been given to us." Our hope is in our unfailing God and his unfailing love for us. Second, the Spirit allows us to cry out to God in our suffering. Galatians 4:6 says, "And because you are sons, God has sent the Spirit of his Son into our hearts, crying, 'Abba! Father!'" God's Spirit dwells in us and proves that we belong to him as children. Third, the Spirit fills us with joy and peace. Romans 15:13 says, "May the God of hope fill you with all joy and peace in believing, so that by the power of the Holy Spirit you may abound in hope."

On my darkest days, it was God's Spirit who breathed hope, joy, and peace into my heart. He brought to mind the Scriptures that were buried in my memory and applied the promises of God to my pain. It was only by his power that I could cling to hope at all, much less abound in it! Yet I found this promise to be true: the Lord was faithful to fill me with the hope that comes only by his Spirit at work in our lives.

Apart from the Lord, our suffering has no purpose and we are without hope. But if our suffering comes to us filtered through the hands of a Father who loves us, we know we can bear it in his strength. If one day our suffering will end and we will enjoy eternity with him in heaven, we know we can endure this temporary pain. If a reigning King will use our suffering to bring about his purposes, we can find joy and peace in the midst of our heartbreak. It is by the power of the Holy Spirit that we abound in hope in our suffering, because he reminds us of these truths. The Spirit applies the balm of God's Word to our wounded hearts (see 1 Cor. 2:12–13).

How God Uses Our Suffering

Although God hates suffering, he is not surprised by it or powerless against it. He is sovereign over all. In his sovereignty, he uses suffering for his glory and for our good.

Our suffering is for God's glory.

In October 2010, I sat in a Bible Study Fellowship lecture, scribbling down notes as fast as I could. Our leader, Julia Robinson, was teaching on Isaiah 7:4: "Be careful, be quiet, do not fear, and do not let your heart be faint." I sat there with a lump in my breast and a biopsy scheduled a few days later. Our leader talked about how we have been spared from the greatest suffering: separation from God. That is all we truly have to fear in this life. All other suffering is temporary, and it will be remedied and redeemed.

And so, our leader argued, because of our salvation in Christ, we have nothing else to fear. We can face suffering in our lives with courage, knowing that God is with us. She exhorted us to take this Christ-centered approach to suffering so that a watching world would see what the Lord has done in our lives and would give him glory. I went home that night and told my husband that if the lump turned out to be cancer, I was ready to suffer for God's glory.

Your friend's cancer diagnosis comes with a challenging assignment: to glorify God by walking with him through suffering. If she belongs to Christ, his mercy and grace will be poured out on her according to her needs, enabling her to endure suffering with Christ's joy and peace (see 2 Cor. 12:9; Phil. 4:19). You have a front-row seat to see how God is sustaining her, and it will be beautiful to watch.

I experienced God's sustaining power and grace even before I heard I had cancer. I can see how God spent years preparing me for this trial. After receiving the diagnosis, I was scared, but I knew that God's Spirit was with me. He worked in my heart to cause me to praise his name during my suffering. I wasn't thankful for cancer, but I was grateful for the opportunity to bring glory to my Redeemer.

Our suffering is for our good.

God's children benefit from suffering. Yes, you read that right. Cancer is not good. But I've seen firsthand how God uses it to accomplish good in the lives of his children. Suffering sanctified me, assured me, and centered me.

Tim Keller says, "Trials and troubles in life, which are inevitable, will either make you or break you. But either way, you will not remain the same."[2] As God was healing me of cancer, he was also healing me of my need for control, selfishness, and fearfulness. I still have a long way to go in each of these areas, but walking through a trial can be a crash-course in sanctification. Joni Eareckson Tada summarizes it this way:

> In short, one form of evil—suffering—is turned on its head to defeat another form of evil—my sin—all to the praise of God's wisdom and glory! Is the cost too great? Is the price of pain too high? Not when you consider that "this light momentary affliction is preparing for us an eternal weight of glory beyond all comparison" (2 Cor. 4:17).[3]

Suffering also led to assurance of my salvation. Before cancer, I sometimes wondered if I truly belonged to Christ or if I just knew all the right answers. In the days following my diagnosis, I knew that my response was due to the Holy Spirit at work in me and not because of my own strength. God filled me with renewed confidence in my salvation and certainty that his Spirit lives in me. Romans 8:9–10 says,

> You, however, are not in the flesh but in the Spirit, if in fact the Spirit of God dwells in you. Anyone who does not have the Spirit of Christ does not belong to him. But if Christ is in you, although the body is dead because of sin, the Spirit is life because of righteousness.

This assurance is a gift from the Lord, as demonstrated by this quote from C. H. Spurgeon: "I mean this, that it is as great a mercy to have your salvation proved to you under trial as it is to have it sustained in you by the consolations of the Spirit of God."[4]

I'm more convinced of the truth of God's character because of my suffering. I have seen how he provides for our needs in difficult circumstances, even when we doubt. I've experienced his peace in an emotional storm. I have watched as he put his faithfulness on display in my life over and over again, in both good and bad circumstances. He is good; he is faithful; he is sovereign. My confidence in these truths helps me to face an uncertain future without despair.

I have seen how suffering makes joy sweeter. The cliché is true: every day is precious, and I'm more aware of it because of the hardship I've endured. Not only is joy in this life sweeter, but I expect we will all find that our joy in heaven will be magnified by our having endured life in this broken world. As Tim Keller says,

> Isn't it possible that the eventual glory and joy we will know will be infinitely greater than it would have been had there been no evil? What if that future world will somehow be greater for having once been broken and lost? If such is the case, that would truly mean the utter defeat of evil. Evil would not just be an obstacle to our beauty and bliss, but it will have only made it better. Evil would have accomplished the very opposite of what it intended.[5]

Only God can turn evil on its head. Only the Almighty can thwart the enemy's purposes by using suffering for good in the lives of God's children. As he weaves pain into a tapestry of beauty for his people, God demonstrates his authority and victory over evil.

How We Walk with God through Suffering

Our trials are painful despite what we know to be true about the Lord, his presence with us in suffering, and his purpose in our suffering. Even when the truth reigns in our minds, sorrow remains in our hearts. How then do we walk through suffering in light of the truth and in the midst of our pain? Scripture gives us a framework for walking with God through suffering, and I'll highlight just a few points here. For a more thorough treatment of this topic, I suggest any of the books that are referenced throughout this resource.

We rejoice and grieve.

First Peter was written to believers who were suffering. In chapter 1, Peter writes,

> Blessed be the God and Father of our Lord Jesus Christ! According to his great mercy, he has caused us to be born again to a living hope through the resurrection of Jesus Christ from the dead, to an inheritance that is imperishable, undefiled, and unfading, kept in heaven for you, who by God's power are being guarded through faith for a salvation ready to be revealed in the last time. In this you rejoice, though now for a little while, if necessary, you have been grieved by various trials, so that the tested genuineness of your faith—more precious than gold that perishes though it is tested by fire—may be found to result in praise and glory and honor at the revelation of Jesus Christ. (vv. 3–7)

We see two responses in these verses that seem contradictory: rejoicing and grieving. Both are ongoing, present realities. The recipients of this letter are suffering, and Peter acknowledges that they are grieved by their troubles. And yet he reminds them to rejoice in God's great mercy, the living hope of Christ, and their eternal, heavenly inheritance. He doesn't tell them to stop grieving so they can rejoice. He exhorts them to rejoice *and* grieve.

When we understand that God hates cancer, it frees us to grieve the effects of cancer. Sometimes we think we should be super-Christians who welcome suffering with enthusiasm. Or we equate joy with a stiff upper lip. But faith in God's sovereignty and goodness goes hand in hand with crying out to him in our distress and sorrow. We find our hope and our joy in Christ, but we still grieve what we lost to cancer. As Keller explains, "[Peter] does not say that we can either rejoice in Christ *or* wail and cry out in pain, but that we can't do both. No, not only can we do both, we *must* do both if we are to grow through our suffering rather than be wrecked by it."[6]

We trust and obey.

Later in Peter's first epistle, we find more about how to walk through suffering. In chapter 4, he writes,

> Beloved, do not be surprised at the fiery trial when it comes upon you to test you, as though something strange were happening to you. But rejoice insofar as you share Christ's sufferings, that you may also rejoice and be glad when his glory is revealed. . . . Therefore let those who suffer according to God's will entrust their souls to a faithful Creator while doing good. (vv. 12–13, 19)

In these verses, we see several responses to suffering that are encouraged by Peter. First, we shouldn't be surprised when we encounter trials. Just as Christ suffered, we should expect to share in his suffering, because we are in him. Second, we are to rejoice, because we know that our suffering brings glory to God. Third, we are to trust our faithful heavenly Father. Finally, we are to continue to do good in the midst of trials.

Trusting God through a trial is challenging. But when we understand the truth of God's character, our faith isn't blind faith. It isn't sugar-coating or denying the pain of our suffering. It is an abiding trust in the sovereign goodness of God in all circumstances, even the ones we cannot understand. Os Guinness puts it this way: "Christians do not say, 'I do not understand you at all, but I trust you anyway.' Rather we say, 'I do not understand you *in this situation*, but I *understand why I trust you anyway.* Therefore I can trust that you understand even though I don't.'"[7] This is the cry of our hearts in suffering: "Lord, I don't understand this, but I believe that you do."

This trust allows us to walk purposefully through suffering, putting one foot in front of the other in obedience to the Lord. Some days we may obey by striking up a conversation with the person next to us in the hospital waiting room. Other days we obey by lying in bed and crying to the Lord in our pain. Our trust and obedience will be imperfect. We will doubt and struggle when we don't understand God's purposes. But his strength is magnified in our weakness. His grace is sufficient for our failure to obey as well as our failure to trust. Through it all, we keep "looking to Jesus, the founder and perfecter of our faith, who for the joy that was set before him endured the cross" as we "run with endurance the race that is set before us" (Heb. 12:1–2).

When I battled cancer, I received many encouraging guestbook messages on the website where I posted updates. But there's one that stood out, and I remember it to this day. It said, "God knows." When I read those two powerful words, I felt a tangible peace and calm. If I couldn't continue standing in strength through the pressure and pain of suffering, God would see my every tear. I didn't need to fear. I didn't need to wonder how it would all turn out. God knows. The one who placed each star in the sky—he knows. The one who gave his Son to rescue me and conquer the evil he hates—he knows. The one who lovingly comforts my loved ones and me—he knows. He knows how he will use my suffering for his glory and for my good. As I suffer or watch those I love endure hardship, I can rejoice and grieve, trust and obey, because God knows.

Questions for Reflection

1. In what ways did this resource challenge your thinking about God's role in our suffering?
2. What are some ways you've seen God use suffering in your life for his glory and/or your good?
3. What do you think it will look like for you to grieve, rejoice, trust, and obey as you watch your friend suffer?

Resource 4.1

Verses to Share with Your Friend

Hope

You make known to me the path of life;
    in your presence there is fullness of joy;
    at your right hand are pleasures forevermore. (Ps. 16:11)

As a deer pants for flowing streams,
    so pants my soul for you, O God.
My soul thirsts for God,
    for the living God.
When shall I come and appear before God?

. . . .

Why are you cast down, O my soul,
    and why are you in turmoil within me?
Hope in God; for I shall again praise him,
    my salvation. (Ps. 42:1–2, 5)

Whom have I in heaven but you?
    And there is nothing on earth that I desire besides you.
My flesh and my heart may fail,
    but God is the strength of my heart and my portion for-
        ever. (Ps. 73:25–26)

Bless the LORD, O my soul,
    and all that is within me,
    bless his holy name!

Bless the LORD, O my soul,
    and forget not all his benefits,
who forgives all your iniquity,
    who heals all your diseases,
who redeems your life from the pit,
    who crowns you with steadfast love and mercy,
who satisfies you with good
    so that your youth is renewed like the eagle's.
        (Ps. 103:1–5)

May the God of hope fill you with all joy and peace in believing, so that by the power of the Holy Spirit you may abound in hope. (Rom. 15:13)

Little children, you are from God and have overcome them, for he who is in you is greater than he who is in the world. (1 John 4:4)

Then I saw a new heaven and a new earth, for the first heaven and the first earth had passed away, and the sea was no more. And I saw the holy city, new Jerusalem, coming down out of heaven from God, prepared as a bride adorned for her husband. And I heard a loud voice from the throne saying, "Behold, the dwelling place of God is with man. He will dwell with them, and they will be his people, and God himself will be with them as their God. He will wipe away every tear from their eyes, and death shall be no more, neither shall there be mourning, nor crying, nor pain anymore, for the former things have passed away."

And he who was seated on the throne said, "Behold, I am making all things new." Also he said, "Write this down, for these words are trustworthy and true." (Rev. 21:1–5)

Peace

Cast your burden on the LORD,
    and he will sustain you;
he will never permit
    the righteous to be moved. (Ps. 55:22)

He is not afraid of bad news;
    his heart is firm, trusting in the LORD.
His heart is steady; he will not be afraid,
    until he looks in triumph on his adversaries.
        (Ps. 112:7–8)

You keep him in perfect peace
    whose mind is stayed on you,
    because he trusts in you.
Trust in the LORD forever,
    for the LORD GOD is an everlasting rock. (Isa. 26:3–4)

But now thus says the LORD,
he who created you, O Jacob,
    he who formed you, O Israel:
"Fear not, for I have redeemed you;
    I have called you by name, you are mine.
When you pass through the waters, I will be with you;
    and through the rivers, they shall not overwhelm you;
when you walk through fire you shall not be burned,
    and the flame shall not consume you." (Isa. 43:1–2)

Peace I leave with you; my peace I give to you. Not as the world gives do I give to you. Let not your hearts be troubled, neither let them be afraid. (John 14:27)

I have said these things to you, that in me you may have peace. In the world you will have tribulation. But take heart; I have overcome the world. (John 16:33)

Do not be anxious about anything, but in everything by prayer and supplication with thanksgiving let your requests be made known to God. And the peace of God, which surpasses all understanding, will guard your hearts and your minds in Christ Jesus. (Phil. 4:6–7)

Love and Care

The LORD is near to the brokenhearted
 and saves the crushed in spirit. (Ps. 34:18)

You have kept count of my tossings;
 put my tears in your bottle.
 Are they not in your book?
Then my enemies will turn back
 in the day when I call.
 This I know, that God is for me.
In God, whose word I praise,
 in the LORD, whose word I praise,
in God I trust; I shall not be afraid.
 What can man do to me? (Ps. 56:8–11)

O God, you are my God; earnestly I seek you;
 my soul thirsts for you;
my flesh faints for you,
 as in a dry and weary land where there is no water.
So I have looked upon you in the sanctuary,
 beholding your power and glory.
Because your steadfast love is better than life,
 my lips will praise you.

So I will bless you as long as I live;
    in your name I will lift up my hands.

My soul will be satisfied as with fat and rich food,
    and my mouth will praise you with joyful lips,
when I remember you upon my bed,
    and meditate on you in the watches of the night;
for you have been my help,
    and in the shadow of your wings I will sing for joy.
My soul clings to you;
    your right hand upholds me. (Ps. 63:1–8)

I have loved you with an everlasting love;
    therefore I have continued my faithfulness to you.
        (Jer. 31:3)

The steadfast love of the LORD never ceases;
    his mercies never come to an end;
they are new every morning;
    great is your faithfulness. (Lam. 3:22–23)

The LORD your God is in your midst,
    a mighty one who will save;
he will rejoice over you with gladness;
    he will quiet you by his love;
he will exult over you with loud singing. (Zeph. 3:17)

Why, even the hairs of your head are all numbered. Fear not;
you are of more value than many sparrows. (Luke 12:7)

No, in all these things we are more than conquerors through
him who loved us. For I am sure that neither death nor life,
nor angels nor rulers, nor things present nor things to come,
nor powers, nor height nor depth, nor anything else in all

creation, will be able to separate us from the love of God in Christ Jesus our Lord. (Rom. 8:37–39)

And my God will supply every need of yours according to his riches in glory in Christ Jesus. (Phil. 4:19)

Refuge

This God—his way is perfect;
    the word of the LORD proves true;
    he is a shield for all those who take refuge in him.
        (Ps. 18:30)

God is our refuge and strength,
    a very present help in trouble.
Therefore we will not fear though the earth gives way,
    though the mountains be moved into the heart of the sea.
        (Ps. 46:1–2)

"Be still, and know that I am God.
    I will be exalted among the nations,
    I will be exalted in the earth!"
The LORD of hosts is with us;
    the God of Jacob is our fortress. (Ps. 46:10–11)

For God alone my soul waits in silence;
    from him comes my salvation.
He alone is my rock and my salvation,
    my fortress; I shall not be greatly shaken. (Ps. 62:1–2)

The LORD is good,
    a stronghold in the day of trouble;
he knows those who take refuge in him. (Nah. 1:7)

Strength

"O our God, will you not execute judgment on them? For we are powerless against this great horde that is coming against us. We do not know what to do, but our eyes are on you."

... And he said, "Listen, all Judah and inhabitants of Jerusalem and King Jehoshaphat: Thus says the LORD to you, 'Do not be afraid and do not be dismayed at this great horde, for the battle is not yours but God's.'" (2 Chron. 20:12, 15)

The LORD is my light and my salvation;
   whom shall I fear?
The LORD is the stronghold of my life;
   of whom shall I be afraid? (Ps. 27:1)

I lift up my eyes to the hills.
   From where does my help come?
My help comes from the LORD,
   who made heaven and earth. (Ps. 121:1–2)

He gives power to the faint,
   and to him who has no might he increases strength.
Even youths shall faint and be weary,
   and young men shall fall exhausted;
but they who wait for the LORD shall renew their strength;
   they shall mount up with wings like eagles;
they shall run and not be weary;
   they shall walk and not faint. (Isa. 40:29–31)

Fear not, for I am with you;
   be not dismayed, for I am your God;
I will strengthen you, I will help you,
   I will uphold you with my righteous right hand. (Isa. 41:10)

But he said to me, "My grace is sufficient for you, for my power is made perfect in weakness." Therefore I will boast all the more gladly of my weaknesses, so that the power of Christ may rest upon me. For the sake of Christ, then, I am content with weaknesses, insults, hardships, persecutions, and calamities. For when I am weak, then I am strong. (2 Cor. 12:9–10)

I can do all things through him who strengthens me. (Phil. 4:13)

Putting Ideas into Action

Use this resource to brainstorm ways you can support your friend and break down the steps you need to take, such as recruiting friends to help, gathering information, or setting aside time to serve her.

Idea	Action Steps
	1.
	2.
	3.
Idea	**Action Steps**
	1.
	2.
	3.

Idea	Action Steps
	1.
	2.
	3.

Idea	Action Steps
	1.
	2.
	3.

Idea	Action Steps
	1.
	2.
	3.

List of Your Friend's Doctors and Nurses

Use this list to keep track of the medical professionals who are working with your friend, both for prayer and for conversation.

Name	Role

Resource 7.1

Calendar Coordination

Here's a place for you to think through your schedule and your friend's schedule, look for places they overlap, and decide if there are any regular commitments you can make to help her logistically.

Regular commitments you can make:

MORNING	You	Her
Sunday		
Monday		
Tuesday		
Wednesday		
Thursday		
Friday		
Saturday		

Calendar Coordination

AFTERNOON	You	Her
Sunday		
Monday		
Tuesday		
Wednesday		
Thursday		
Friday		
Saturday		

EVENING	You	Her
Sunday		
Monday		
Tuesday		
Wednesday		
Thursday		
Friday		
Saturday		

Seasonal Plans

You can use this list to brainstorm seasonal needs your friend has and ways you can plan to help (or recruit others to help).

Spring

Birthdays or anniversaries?

Holiday help?

Change closets?

Spring clean?

Summer

Birthdays or anniversaries?

Holiday help?

Fall

Birthdays or anniversaries?

Holiday help?

Change closets?

Back to school?

Flu season?

Winter

Birthdays or anniversaries?

Holiday help?

Flu season?

Resource 7.3

Meal Plans

This is a place to make notes about meals you plan to take to your friend, her dislikes, and her preferences.

Date	Meal

Dietary restrictions or dislikes:

Favorite recipes:

Resource 10.1

Prayer Plan

Use this resource to keep track of prayer requests your friend shares and your prayers for her.

Date	Prayer

Notes

Chapter Three: When the Going Gets Tough

1. Kara Tippetts and Jill Lynn Buteyn, *Just Show Up: The Dance of Walking through Suffering Together* (Colorado Springs: David C. Cook, 2015), 157–58.

Chapter Four: When Religious Platitudes Fail You

1. Dietrich Bonhoeffer, *Life Together*, trans. John W. Doberstein (New York: HarperOne, 1954), 97–98.
2. Kara Tippetts and Jill Lynn Buteyn, *Just Show Up: The Dance of Walking Through Suffering Together* (Colorado Springs: David C. Cook, 2015), 10.
3. Ibid., 64.

Chapter Five: Diagnosis

1. A port is a small medical device surgically placed right under the skin, typically near the collarbone, that is used to administer intravenous chemotherapy.

Chapter Nine: Mind

1. See Question 1 of the Westminster Shorter Catechism.

Chapter Ten: Soul

1. First Corinthians 10:13 says that you will not be tempted beyond what you can bear, because God will provide a way out. But this

verse about sin and temptation often gets twisted around and incorrectly used to refer to suffering.

Resource 2.1: A Biblical View of Community

1. Dietrich Bonhoeffer, *Life Together*, trans. John W. Doberstein (New York: HarperOne, 1954), 18.
2. Adam S. McHugh, *The Listening Life: Embracing Attentiveness in a World of Distraction* (Downers Grove, IL: InterVarsity Press, 2015), 162.
3. Timothy Keller, *Walking with God through Pain and Suffering* (New York: Riverhead Books, 2015), 193.
4. Bonhoeffer, *Life Together*, 23.
5. Dave Furman, *Being There: How to Love Those Who Are Hurting* (Wheaton, IL: Crossway, 2016), 62.
6. See Bonhoeffer, *Life Together*, 23.
7. James Morwood, ed., *Pocket Oxford Latin Dictionary*, 3rd ed. (Oxford: Oxford University Press, 2005), s.v. "communitas."

Resource 3.1: A Biblical View of Suffering

1. Timothy Keller, *Walking with God through Pain and Suffering* (New York: Penguin Books, 2015), 121.
2. Ibid., 190.
3. Joni Eareckson Tada, "God's Plan A," in *Be Still, My Soul: Embracing God's Purpose and Provision in Suffering*, ed. Nancy Guthrie (Wheaton, IL: Crossway, 2010), 35.
4. Charles Haddon Spurgeon, "Faith Tried and Proved," in ibid., 103–4.
5. Keller, *Walking with God*, 117.
6. Ibid., 252.
7. Os Guinness, "When We Don't Know Why, We Trust God Who Knows Why," in Guthrie, *Be Still, My Soul*, 38.

For Further Reading

Bonhoeffer, Dietrich. *Life Together*. Translated by John W. Dober-stein. New York: HarperOne, 1954. [A classic work on the nature of Christian community.]

Furman, Dave. *Being There: How to Love Those Who Are Hurting*. Wheaton, IL: Crossway, 2016. [A pastoral, practical book about how to be a friend to someone who's suffering.]

Guthrie, Nancy, ed. *Be Still, My Soul: Embracing God's Purpose and Provision in Suffering*. Wheaton, IL: Crossway, 2010. [A collection of readings from various authors, pastors, and theologians on the topics of suffering, purpose, and hope.]

Guthrie, Nancy. *Hearing Jesus Speak into Your Sorrow*. Carol Stream, IL: Tyndale, 2009. [A book about grief and trusting Jesus in your pain.]

Keller, Timothy. *Walking with God through Pain and Suffering*. New York: Riverhead Books, 2015. [A comprehensive book about suffering in our culture and in the Bible.]

Silk, Susan, and Barry Goldman. "How Not to Say the Wrong Thing." *Los Angeles Times*, April 7, 2013. http://www.latimes.com/nation /la-oe-0407-silk-ring-theory-20130407-story.html. [A valuable article that describes how to support your friend and not burden her with your feelings.]

Sullivan, Marilyn. *A Patch of Comfort*. Mustang, OK: Tate Publishing, 2011. [A short book about what grief feels like and how to support a grieving friend.]

Tada, Joni Eareckson. *A Place of Healing: Wrestling with the Mysteries of Suffering, Pain, and God's Sovereignty*. Colorado Springs: David C. Cook, 2010. [A book to help with developing a biblical view of suffering and God's character.]

Tippetts, Kara. *The Hardest Peace: Expecting Grace in the Midst of Life's Hard*. Colorado Springs: David C. Cook, 2014. [A young mother's story of trusting God in the struggle of incurable cancer.]

Tippetts, Kara, and Jill Lynn Buteyn. *Just Show Up: The Dance of Walking through Suffering Together*. Colorado Springs: David C. Cook, 2015. [The story of a community surrounding a young mother with incurable cancer.]

Index of Subjects and Names